DOCTOR'S NINE-MONTH RIVAL

KRISTINE LYNN

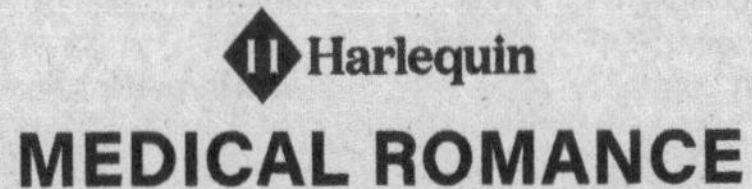

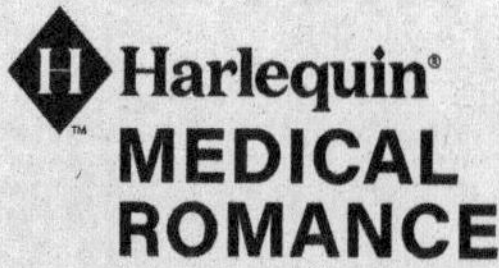

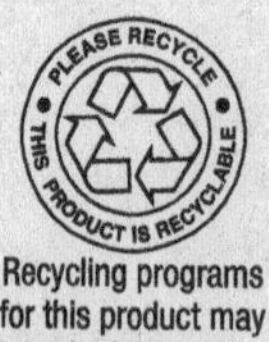

Recycling programs for this product may not exist in your area.

ISBN-13: 978-1-335-99366-3

Doctor's Nine-Month Rival

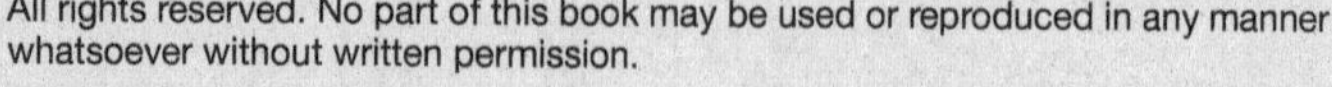

For questions and comments about the quality of this book, please contact us at CustomerService@Harlequin.com.

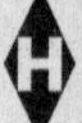

Harlequin Enterprises ULC
22 Adelaide St. West, 41st Floor
Toronto, Ontario M5H 4E3, Canada
www.Harlequin.com

HarperCollins Publishers
Macken House, 39/40 Mayor Street Upper,
Dublin 1, D01 C9W8, Ireland
www.HarperCollins.com

Printed in U.S.A.

1 2 3 4 5 6 7 8 9 10 HDC 28 27 26 25

Paging Dr. Morrison

*One hospital, two doctor brothers—
and two one-night surprises!*

Mack and Rhett Morrison might look alike, might both be skilled trauma docs, and might be about to find themselves working in the same Austin ER... but that's where the similarities end. Raised by a careless father, both sons have striven to distance themselves from his influence and each other.

Mack is the steady, responsible Head of ER. Rhett has lived life on the edge as an F1 Medic, until he returns to Texas. But when a single night changes both their lives forever, the brothers must face the consequences—and fatherhood—at the same time!

In *Expecting in the ER*

Lainey has returned to Austin Memorial with shocking news for her ex-husband. Their one unplanned night of passion had consequences, and she now has a job in Mack Morrison's ER. Will the secret she's keeping tear down the walls between them, or finally tear them apart?

In *Doctor's Nine-Month Rival*

Dr. Rhett Morrison thrives on dangerous pursuits, and competing with Dr. Jacqueline Elliot for a coveted post at Austin Memorial is his toughest challenge yet! For Jacqueline turns out to be the stranger he shared one passionate night with—and she's carrying his baby!

Both available now!

Dear Reader,

Welcome to Austin Memorial and book two in a duet about the Morrison brothers and their path to redemption—with their pasts, insecurities and barriers to love.

When Jack meets Rhett in a bar the night before her first day at a new job, how is she to know he's the brother to her future boss—and that their tryst will lead to an accidental pregnancy? Or that a month later, they'll be pitted against one another for the same position at the hospital!

The tension that follows as these two fight for not only their place in Austin Memorial Hospital, but one another's hearts, is palpable. In this forced-proximity, rivals-to-lovers, accidental-pregnancy story, the only thing on the line besides patients' lives are the hearts of these two doctors.

This duet was so much fun to write, especially with Tina's characters, Mack and Lainey, as strong supports. If you haven't checked out book one in this duet, you definitely should!

Enjoy these two books and let me know your thoughts on Jack and Rhett, and their path to love. Drop me a line on X, Instagram or Facebook, or by email at kristinelynnauthor@gmail.com.

Thanks for reading!

XO, *Kristine*

Hopelessly addicted to espresso and HEAs, **Kristine Lynn** pens high-stakes romances in the wee morning hours before teaching writing at an Oregon college. Luckily, the stakes there aren't as dire. When she's not grading, writing, or searching for the perfect vanilla latte, she can be found on the hiking trails behind her home with her daughter and puppy. She'd love to connect on X, Facebook, or Instagram.

Books by Kristine Lynn

Harlequin Medical Romance

Royal York Hospital

Wedding Date with Dr. Petrides

Brought Together by His Baby
Accidentally Dating His Boss
Their Six-Month Marriage Ruse
A Kiss with the Irish Surgeon
Nine Months to Marry the Princess
How to Resist Your Enemy

Visit the Author Profile page at Harlequin.com.

For The Fab Five, my soul/sole sisters

Our shared love of books, deep talks, runs, swims and wine dates are the motivation to do the rest of life, especially when it's hard. Thank you for all the miles.

PROLOGUE

Dr. Everett Morrison assessed the situation. He didn't like it, not one bit. He worried his bottom lip as he sutured the three-inch gash on his patient's forehead.

"This is messy," he said to no one in particular. To his patient, he added, "But the scar won't even show in two months."

"You're that good, Doc?" Federico asked. He was the lead F1 driver for the team of racers Everett was attached to, along with other medical personnel.

"I'm that good." He winked and stepped back to admire his work. Efficient, quick and clean. No one would accuse him of being sloppy, with medicine at least.

"Can I still drive?" Federico asked.

Everett winced. That was the million-dollar question, wasn't it? Or rather the $5.2 million question if Federico won the circuit. Only three more races determined the outcome for their team, and this driver was their best bet for finishing strong. They couldn't afford not to race Federico, but could Federico handle the pressure on his wound when he was hitting close to 5 g's on the first turn?

The car was damaged, but that wasn't Everett's circus to wrangle—he'd leave that up to the pit crew.

"How's the car?" he asked in his earpiece. Static crackled in his ear.

"Good as it can be. She'll run, but he's gotta be careful around the first two turns."

Everett pinched the bridge of his nose. *Fuck.* He didn't want to make this call. By far, this was the worst accident he'd seen someone walk away from, and Federico had escaped almost unscathed, the slice to his forehead all he had to show for the disaster.

In medical terms, he was on borrowed time.

"What'd they say?" he asked Everett.

"Car'll run. But that's not my concern. You are."

There were thirty-two ways this could go wrong, and only one that landed the team safely on the other side. A perfect run. And perfect wasn't possible out there. The only thing that was?

Danger. Risk. Peril.

But wasn't that the perk of what Everett did for a living? Mitigate and understand medical risk in arenas where danger was literally around every corner?

"I can do it, Doc. You've watched me race with sprains, migraines and worse."

Pride warmed his chest, pushed out the doubt. Federico was right. Not only had Everett seen him race through hellish conditions and pull his team to win after win, he'd made sure they were safe doing it.

Everett loved the thrill of being a traveling doctor, attached to high-risk patients whose lives were in the balance every time they stepped into their arena—rodeos, races and rock faces. He lived for the adrenaline rush. Lived for it the same way Federico and the other racers lived to drive.

Federico's face was stoic, unreadable, except to Everett. He could see the tic in the racer's jaw, the one that betrayed how much hinged on Everett's answer.

That, he understood. If someone tried to take this life from him, he'd rage and burn down whatever stood in his way.

"Let's make sure the wound can withstand the pressure on turn one."

"Yes. Thanks, Doc."

Everett placed a bandage over the wound, securing it with medical tape. That was only step one.

"It's gonna hurt. You sure you wanna do this?"

The fire in Federico's eyes would have been answer enough, but he kept his gaze pinned to Everett's as the racer's head was fitted with a gauze bandage over the other one that was there. His teeth were gritted.

"Absolutely. You know it'll kill me if I don't."

Everett ignored his very real fear—that it might kill Federico if he *did*. That wasn't his call. All he could control was making sure his patients were aware of the risks and set them up with the best medical care he could offer.

As an amateur racer himself, and adrenaline junkie to boot, Everett "Rhett" Morrison knew the dangers inherent in adventure sports like Formula 1 racing. He'd loved practicing medicine since the first time he got ahold of his brother's stethoscope, but car racing, bull riding and rock climbing were how he felt *alive*.

Still, doing it as a career where the stakes were so much higher was a different beast. It clouded drivers' vision, gave a number of them a false sense of immunity to the dangers when the purse was as high as it was.

But explaining that wasn't his job. They had a team psychologist who traveled with them, and that was the last gig Everett wanted. Not when so much was at stake with a driver's mental capacity to withstand the stress of the race.

Nah. Give him literal injuries any day of the

week—wounds he could see and heal. And that's what he'd done.

He stepped back once more to appraise his work. "It'll hold. Rest is up to you, kid."

Federico's smile was wide, even if it boasted a split top lip that made the whole scene a bit macabre.

"Catch ya on the flipside, Doc." He turned back just as he got to the car, which looked as worn as its driver. "And thanks. This means everything to me."

"Just drive safe," Everett said, waving Federico on. The kid was like a labradoodle, all fluff and play. In some ways he was perfect for this sport. The racer took off on the track, the speed building as he drove out of sight. Everett hated this course for how limited the viewing was.

That, and the deadly hairpin on turn one.

He kept his gaze fixed on the screen highlighting the race from a bird's-eye view. Federico made it into turn two. Only then did Everett exhale. One thing he hadn't considered when he took on this unconventional medical career was how the stress would play out on his own body as he grew to know and care for his clients. It wasn't like the ER where patients came in and out through the revolving door, never staying long. They either healed or...didn't.

On the rodeo or F1 circuit, however, Everett's

job was to stay with a team for the season, keeping them healthy and prepared for the strain of what the months of endurance would demand of him—or her.

It was high octane in more than one way, and Everett loved it for all the reasons his brother Mack hated that life. It was fast, dangerous and just reckless enough that it staved off the pervasive feelings of self-inflicted loneliness. Everett's prescription for an emotionally avoidant father and generational trauma from that particular relationship was running away from anything resembling a life his dad would have chosen for him. That meant fast as hell race cars and horses.

Mack, also a physician, chose the calmer, safer route. He did everything he could to be the man their dad hadn't been—stable, solid and reliable. His medical career at a hospital in Austin, Texas, was benign, his dating nonexistent since his divorce, his judgment of Everett fierce and all-consuming. In Mack's eyes, Everett was on the road to becoming their dad, even though nothing could be farther from the truth.

Their dad, the coward that he was, pretended to desire a stable, loving home life and thriving business. But in reality, Thom Morrison had a whole life of cheating, in and out of his marriage. There were at least three women who claimed to be in a serious relationship with Thom, and one of them had a daughter she claimed was his.

Which meant Mack and Everett had a sister they barely knew. Thom Morrison was also not the stand-up philanthropic businessman he purported to be. No, he flitted around the world making his billions scamming broken companies into selling their businesses to his firm.

In short, Mack and Everett's dad was an asshole. And the sole reason Everett wasn't going to *pretend* to do anything. He wanted a fast-paced life where no one could claim him as theirs, meaning he couldn't hurt anyone with the genetic probability he'd disappoint them.

It wasn't that he didn't want a family or partner. But those demanded stability and even then, simply choosing someone to share your life didn't guarantee you'd end up with them. What if, like their dad, he couldn't commit? Or what if he did, as he had in college, and she left him in the end anyway, just like Lainey had left Mack? Nah, it was better to only rely on himself. It was cleaner that way.

"You sure he's got this, Rhett?" the medic attached to the team asked, employing Everett's nickname. Everett shook his head out of the fog of his dredged up past.

"Hey, Tony." Tony was a local who didn't travel outside the EU circuit with the core team, but he was an integral part of the crew. His eyes on a situation were usually focused on the blind spots, but what more could Everett have done? "I sure hope so. He's a helluva driver and I stitched him up the best I could."

"I'm not worried about your work, or his driving. I'm more worried his adrenaline will catch up to him and how that'll show up on the course."

"Me, too," Everett agreed. His own chest muscles were tight as the whir and roar of the engines filled the arena where the medical team was stationed. The course was beautiful, winding through some of the wealthiest homes in Barcelona. The air was thick with tension and exhaust, and the thrill-chasing part of Everett's heart thumped a little louder as the racers came back around the track.

Federico was in the lead. His car took the final turn and—

The sound of tires being scraped over asphalt wasn't congruent with the smooth hum of the racers behind the lead car. Like a slow-motion film, the scene played out in flashes.

Federico's car sliding into the turn and losing traction.

The car behind him hitting his bumper, sending him into a spin.

The crushing of metal on metal as a third car slammed into Federico.

The part of Everett that thrived on medicine and healing froze momentarily before springing into action. He grabbed his medical bag and tore out of the tent toward the crash. Three ambulances met him at the mangled car, one of the teams already working to extract Federico from the twisted metal that had once been his car.

"He's ours. I've got this," Everett said, breathless, his heart pounding.

Please be okay, he pleaded with whomever might be listening to errant prayers from desperate doctors.

When they removed Federico from the car, his head injury still wrapped, but new bloodied wounds gaping on his cheeks and chin, Everett gritted his teeth. He didn't think he'd ever forget the scene or smell of burnt metal and flesh.

Then he got to work on saving his patient, a job he'd signed up for and at that moment couldn't remember a single reason why.

Everett walked into the bar jet-lagged and hung over thanks to the three whiskeys he had on the flight back to the States. It wasn't a mystery that he'd picked Austin as his destination. He had family there, even if he still wasn't sure he'd reach out to Mack.

The last thing he needed was an "I told you so."

He also didn't need another whiskey, but until

the image of Federico's face when he woke and found out he'd never walk again was erased from Everett's mind whenever he closed his eyes, this was the only Rx to ease the pain.

"Black Label, neat," he said when the bartender came around. His voice was thick with no sleep and too much…everything. His only thought on the transatlantic flight was whether he'd been going about this all the wrong way.

Still, he had one more contract to fulfill, and he'd asked for it to be transferred to Austin for the final race at the Circuit of the Americas.

Then he'd figure out what to do next. Maybe take time off from the circuits and do a semipermanent stint as a traveling hospitalist. Maybe take an interim position at a hospital in the southwest. He didn't know, but he had time to figure it out.

The drink was placed in front of him, and he didn't sip it like he usually would. No, he shot the whole thing in a single swallow, letting it burn his throat all the way down.

"That kind of reckless consumption of good whiskey is punishable by jail time down here," a voice to his left said. His body reacted viscerally to the smooth sound, chills chasing down his spine and heat pooling low in his abdomen.

Fuck, if a voice could do that—

He smiled, turning to face the snarky comment head-on, and choked on whatever remnant of whiskey was left in his throat. The woman was shorter than him by almost a foot, but with her giant chocolate-brown eyes lined with mascara, she still took up all the space at the bar. Eyes that were peering into his like she could see through every last cell making up his body.

She had an off-center smile, like she was worrying her bottom lip between her teeth, and the heat from his stomach filled his jeans instead. When she draped her long brown curls over her right shoulder, exposing the skin on the left, he temporarily forgot everything—his name, why he was in Austin, whatever trauma had led to the permanent ache in his chest above his heart.

"That right? Well, what can a newcomer do to remedy that?" he asked.

"Don't know you can fix what you already broke," she said, and he felt that in his gut. Didn't he know it… "But you can start by buying another round and taking your time."

He laughed. "Good plan. Does it help my case if I buy the gorgeous woman to my right one as well?"

She shrugged and there was no mistaking it, she bit her bottom lip and aimed that off-kilter smile right at him. When she glanced down at her half-empty glass, he noticed she had a single arrow tattoo along her wrist. It was delicate and stunning, like her.

"I'm not done with the drink I have," she noted.

"You will be if you join me in lawless shooting of good liquor."

She laughed, her head thrown back in joy. Damn, she was alluring.

He took advantage of her lapsed attention to give her a once-over and had to say—the slight, athletically curvy frame poured into black jeans and a sheer black top wasn't doing any other women at the bar any favors. He was more than half hard.

Interesting. One of the perks of not settling down was his ability to have fun when he met a woman interested in the same no-strings brand of entertainment he was. He'd met some lovely, beautiful women during his time as managing physician of a Formula 1 racing team.

But none of them had ever captured his attention so fully at first glance.

He waved the bartender over. "Two more, please. And I'll pick up her tab."

"No," she argued, "I can take care of myself. I made this mess, I'll clean it up." It was his turn to laugh. And be impressed. Not many women turned down his attempt to spoil them.

"Fair enough. I'm Everett. Friends call me Rhett."

She took his outstretched hand, and even though biologically he knew it was bullshit, he'd have sworn he felt heat between their palms when they touched.

"Rhett, hmm? Nice to meet you. I'm Jacqueline. Friends don't call me Jackie, not if they want to live to tell about it."

"What *do* friends call you?" he asked. He leaned in, catching a whiff of her perfume. The spicy citrus scent made his mouth water. Would she taste like she smelled?

Well, that was an idiotic thought. Of course she wouldn't. But he wanted to test the theory either way. What other kind of hold would this woman have over him if he gave in to his very real, very sudden desire to kiss her?

She leaned in as well, taking her fresh glass and clinking it with his.

"I'm not sure I'm ready to tell you that. We just met, after all."

"So, we're not friends? I did buy you a drink, if that helps my cause," he teased. Banter with this woman was fun. Excitement took over where the whiskey left off.

She sipped her drink and licked her lips.

His tingled, wondering what hers would feel like pressed against his.

"You did. But I don't think I can be friends with a man who doesn't appreciate good whiskey and tries to white knight my bar tab."

"Can we sweep it all up under 'chivalry'? I've heard it's not dead in Texas."

She laughed and shook her head. When her hand landed on his forearm, he was 100 percent certain there was a buzz of electricity that time. "Not quite. But I'm not sure I'm looking for friends. I'm here for work, and when I get invested, I take life pretty seriously."

She sounded like his brother, but with the gleam of mischief in her eyes, it was infinitely more appealing on her.

"You have a partner?"

A dark shadow passed over her face and she shook her head. "No. No one." The finality in her statement made him curious, but he hedged and kept his questions tucked away. She was right—they'd just met. Why did he care why she reacted in certain ways to something he said?

"I'm here for work, too. And when I start Friday, I won't have any free time, either. So how about we're *friends* tonight and see where things take us from there? No strings."

His heart thumped an extra beat at that last part. No strings was part of his MO. Condoms and one night only meant no chance he'd accidentally make good on their father's clause to get access to their trust—continuing the family line of Morrisons. Neither him nor Mack wanted their dad's money, not when it came with such seedy parameters.

Too bad he got the feeling he'd need more than just a night with this intriguing woman to appreciate everything she was and brought to the table.

More than a night wasn't possible, though. Not with his history, and not with the uncertainty of his own future staring him down the barrel. Not especially with the pervasive fear he'd done everything he could not to end up like his old man, only to do just that.

His options were limited.

"No strings aren't my thing, normally." He held his hope on the "normally." She bit her lip again and the hope blossomed. "But what do you propose, my new friend, Rhett?"

All the traumatic memories from his past evaporated and nothing could stop the smile that formed on his lips. He took her hand and kissed her knuckles, watching a shade of red paint her cheeks. What a canvas she was…

He wondered, did the blush extend down her chest?

Those were answers he wanted to discover about his new "friend."

"Well, I was thinking you could tell me your favorite dessert, we could find a place in Austin that makes it and go from there."

Where had he drummed that up? He'd come

into the bar to get whiskey drunk and forget the horror show of Federico's crash that still haunted him.

But…in all fairness, the images were gone. For now, at least. It might be a different method that made them disappear, but who was he to argue with the results? Maybe he'd get some rest tonight if this woman's presence kept the nightmares at bay and he could focus on finishing his last three-week contract with the Firestone team and what came next.

"If you can find a bakery open this late that will have a double-thick brownie, I'll not only tell you my nickname, but I'll name my firstborn child after you, Rhett."

He took her hand and left a fifty-dollar bill on the bar. "Challenge accepted," he said.

She rubbed his palm with her thumb, and his body went on high alert. This woman was going to be just the distraction he needed to figure out how he was supposed to continue to practice medicine when his last patient had barely survived. A patient who blamed him and wouldn't return his calls to the hospital to talk.

"Any idea where we should start?" she asked.

He sent her a wicked grin. "If you're willing to wait till the bakery around the corner from my hotel opens at six tomorrow morning, I know just where to start."

He expected a slap across his face from the woman he'd just propositioned without knowing anything other than her first name, but she raised her brows at him and turned that perfect shade of red again.

"I'll accept those terms. But I'm holding you to that brownie."

He led her from the bar, keeping her hand in his.

As they made their way to his hotel, the cool spring air enveloping them, Rhett felt his chest loosen just enough that he could breathe. He didn't know how, couldn't see when, but he felt that things just might be okay. At the very least, he had a beautiful woman on his arm and the possibility of changing his medical career on the horizon.

He ignored the image of his father's face looming in the shadows of his mind. Absently, he felt in his wallet, ensuring he had a condom tucked away in there, just in case.

Besides another whiskey and an "I told you so," an unwanted pregnancy tying Rhett to anyone anywhere was the third last thing he needed.

With that, he opened the door to his hotel, excited for the night ahead, leaving his father, his brother and his last crash patient outside the room.

Tonight was about fun. The rest could wait.

CHAPTER ONE

Four weeks later

EVERETT STOOD OUTSIDE the hospital, ignoring the mid-March Austin wind that whipped around him. The chill was worse with the mist from Lady Bird Lake, but it was the least of his problems.

The first—and much bigger than the weather—was the email from a recruiter he'd given his information to a month ago. The F1 contract had ended, and with no more drama or injury, thank God. He'd had a couple hits on interim positions, as well as substantial offers from both the Austin rodeo circuit and the U.S.-based race team asking to extend his contract. They'd both told him to write a number and they'd give it to him.

The younger version of him from medical school would have jumped at those two offers. Even the version of him that had come from Barcelona wanted to chase that high of exhilaration that only came from the fast-paced world of trauma medicine.

But he hadn't been able to think past the image of Federico being pulled from the car. Sure, it was always a possibility that an accident would happen—more than likely a probability given the sport he chose to practice with. Still, knowing Federico had trusted him with the go-ahead was what ate him up inside, changed his mind about his ability to go back to that kind of medicine. He figured he would eventually, but for now, he needed to get his head right.

So, he'd practice somewhere safe, then make some decisions in six months or so.

Hence the job announcement that was bugging him.

Career opportunity available in your area, the subject line of the email read. Nice. Convenient, too. When Everett opened it, though, all thoughts of safety were off the table.

At first glance, it was perfect. Interim six-month position in the emergency room as a trauma doc. Renewable contract upon completion if the applicant and hospital were both willing to renegotiate the terms. A salary that rivaled what he'd been making as a contractor.

There was one nonnegotiable caveat, however.

His brother, Mack, would be his supervisor.

Yeah, that wasn't going to work. He and Mack were estranged to say the least. It wasn't as if some big thing had happened; the two of them were just…different. Everett was, according to Mack, "irresponsible and wasting his talents" on contract medicine. Mack was, according to Everett, "a bore who needed to get laid and a sense of humor, probably in that order."

He wasn't an idiot; he knew why he and Mack were the way they were. They were both products of their father's shitty upbringing, and they were both handling it in very different ways.

Ostensibly, he should walk away from this offer and find anything else anywhere else. How could he expect to calm his nervous system enough to heal if he was around his judgmental brother all day every day?

But it's the only job that's cropped up in Austin.

Which led to his second problem. Everett hadn't been able to forget the woman he'd brought back to his hotel room on his first night in town. *Jacqueline.* That one word summed up everything he knew about her, save the intangibles—that he still smelled her scent on his jacket from that night, that he still tasted her every time he sipped his morning coffee, that his body still ached for the singular pleasure that was sleeping with her.

They'd shared only one night, but the hours in her arms kissing, touching, pulling and pushing, tasting—all of it—were some of the best he'd ever spent in the company of a woman.

Hell, period.

The nightmares had abated that night and the next, but had come back since. He credited Jacqueline for being one part calm and two parts passion and spice.

Which was why this damned job in Austin was so appealing, despite the other reasons it shouldn't be. He needed to find her again. He'd been back to the bar a dozen times and scoured the parks and restaurants near it.

And nothing. It was like he'd had the best night of his life with a ghost.

It wasn't as if he'd know what to do if he did find her again. He didn't date, couldn't fathom committing to someone, especially now that his life was in limbo, but he also couldn't shake her, which was *weird.*

In part because he hadn't been able to be with anyone since.

Anyway, it didn't matter. If this meeting with his brother went south, which he had every reason to think it would, he'd be leaving Austin and finding the first job that didn't make him question being a trauma doctor.

He walked through the doors to the hospital lobby and inhaled sharply. The foyer was beautiful. Oak-lined ceilings and juxtaposed cerulean and white walls made the entrance look like a swanky hotel lobby, not the gateway to one of the southwest's premier labor and delivery hospitals—and busiest emergency rooms thanks to the rodeo's popularity in Austin.

A woman in pink scrubs walked up to him.

"I'd know that face anywhere. You're Dr. Morrison's brother, aren't you?" she asked. Her smile didn't betray any knowledge of the brothers' fraught relationship. "I'm Julie, the head of Peds."

"Sure am. I'm the other Dr. Morrison, actually. Everett Morrison. Nice to meet you, Julie." He shook her hand. "Any way you could direct me to his office?"

"I'd love to. I'm on my way there anyway to drop off the final rotation for our interns. So, are you just visiting, or planning on joining the team?"

Everett tried on a smile, but knowing he was on his way to see his brother after barely laying eyes on the guy for half a decade at least didn't make it easy. His stomach rolled with anxiety, an unfamiliar feeling. He should have had breakfast.

"We'll see. I'm not sure if the job's been taken, but I'd like to find out more about it either way."

She led him down a well-lit corridor with artistic photos of children in various stages of what looked like cancer treatment. He stopped to look at one. Next to the photos were paragraphs about the children and a piece of art they'd drawn while they were in long-term care at Austin Memorial.

"These are," he started. Everett swallowed, but his throat was dry. "These are touching."

"It was your brother's idea, actually. The kids love seeing their faces up on the wall. They say it makes them feel famous."

Everett let out a humorless chuckle. "That's actually kind of cute." But…when did Mack start thinking about kids and stuff like that? What he didn't know about his older sibling could fill every bed in this hospital.

"Anyway, you're the second person in two days to put your name in for the interim position, which is kind of exciting."

"Oh yeah? Has it been posted long?"

Julie shook her head. "Nope. Six days. The other candidate did some hospitalist work for us the past month, but is looking for something more stable. Between you two, we shouldn't need more candidates, though. You're both super qualified."

Everett frowned. He'd been unsure whether he wanted to work with his brother, but hadn't even considered that Mack wouldn't choose him for the job if he outright asked for it.

Of course he wouldn't. You two have barely spoken in years.

Yeah, but he'd made the effort to reach out, to set up this appointment. He'd make sure his brother knew he was serious in honoring at least a six-month contract. That was all Mack had wanted from him at one point.

Needless to say, by the time they turned the corner, Everett was even less certain about being there than when he'd walked in.

"So, what do you know about the other candidate?" he asked. Maybe he could regain some confidence by sussing out his competition. At the least, Everett was damned good at his job.

Julie smiled. "Jack Elliot. Helluva doctor and equally good with kids. Was CMO of a hospital on the east coast, I think. Somewhere near Boston."

Damn. That was impressive. Something Mack would love.

"Nice," was all he could muster. Then they were at his brother's office door, an impressive sign boasting acronyms next to Mack's name. "Well, thanks, Julie. It was really nice meeting you. I hope we'll have a chance to work together."

"Me, too. Good luck, other Dr. Morrison."

From the sounds of it, he'd need it.

He went to knock—an odd concept for seeing family, but somehow it seemed appropriate—when the door opened.

His body was aware of several things at the same time. The scent of citrus and spice, the wave of espresso curls cascading over a shoulder draped in a black satin blouse, the lilt of a thick, sensual voice as it called out, "Thanks, Dr. Morrison."

And then there were the eyes that had haunted him for almost a month staring up at him, wide with surprise. He waited a beat, then a smile formed beneath them. For the first time in four weeks, Everett exhaled.

Jacqueline.

"I've been looking everywhere for you," he said. Instantly, he regretted it. He sounded like a low-grade stalker.

"Rhett," she whispered. She shook her head and smiled, and he realized how much he'd missed her grin. "It's good to see you."

"Uh, yeah. You, too. Strange, but good."

"Out of curiosity, where did you look for me?"

"The bar, the shops and food joints near it…everywhere I thought you might be. I guess I sound like an idiot since we made the 'one night friendship' rule, but I kinda wanted to see you again."

"I feel the same. It was…nice to spend that time with you and yeah, maybe in another world, we could've had more fun as friends," she said, that last word something of an inside joke between them. "But I started work and I really need to concentrate on it. Still, it's good to see you here."

"Same. It's kind of a weird coincidence. I mean, here I am looking for you and just as I was about to give up, I found you as I'm coming to ask for a job. Life's funny, huh?"

He chuckled, but the shadow that he'd seen that

night they'd met when he asked her about a boyfriend or husband passed over her face again.

"The interim trauma doc position?"

He nodded. "How did you—"

"Life's funny, alright. That's why I'm here, too. I was just talking to the boss."

Everett shook his head as reality hit him square across the temple. "You're Jack?"

"Yeah. The name works better for work, for obvious reasons. And you're really here to apply?"

"I am. I'm Rhett Morrison. The other Dr. Morrison, whose brother is the boss."

She let out a laugh devoid of any humor. Her eyes turned almost black and her body went rigid. "Fabulous. So I work here a month learning the ropes and making myself part of the community, only to be put up against the brother of the man in charge of hiring. That seems like my kind of luck." She shook her head and moved past him. The air around them shifted, tension taking the space she'd just inhabited.

"It's not like—" he tried to say. She put up a hand to stop him.

"I know what it's like. Because I've had to earn everything I ever got, from my freedom to jobs, to respect. I've also watched every man I know step into my life and take what he thinks is his regardless of whether he's earned it. Well, not this time. So, Everett Morrison, you can go in there and get all chummy with your brother, but don't think for a second I'm not going to fight you for this job. What happened between us is in the past, and this is my future. There's no chance in hell I'm giving it over to you because we slept together, okay?"

What could Everett do but nod? She'd all but accused him of nepotism and stealing the position out from under her by using his ties to Mack. Which, if he was honest with himself, he was fully prepared to do if "Jack" was anyone other than the woman who'd stolen his attention and infected his thoughts since he'd met her at the bar a month ago.

"Jack, I—"

She whipped around, her curls a sea of dark brown crashing along her chest. "Don't you dare. Only friends can call me that, and I think it's obvious you and I are never going to be friends, Everett. Good luck in there—you're going to need it."

She spun on her heel and only then was he aware of the fact that her icy demeanor did nothing to quelch the desire he felt for the woman. Well, that was inconvenient.

Everett watched her walk away, the oddness of the whole situation settling in. He'd found her, but in the worst way possible. If he got the job, he'd take it from her and who knew if she'd stay in Austin. But if he didn't, he'd have to leave her behind. Both seemed unconscionable.

"Shit," he mumbled. What was he supposed to do? Standing in the hallway wasn't giving him any ideas. "Might as well get this over with."

He knocked on his brother's door and waited until he heard the stoic baritone on the other side.

"Come in," Mack said.

With that, Everett strode through the doorway, coming face-to-face with his past. The question was, how much could he hope that this man—a guy he shared almost 100 percent of his genes with, but couldn't be more different from—would help him on the path to his future?

And why, when he thought of his future, was Jack's face the only thing he saw?

That didn't matter right now. Couldn't matter. He had things to do first.

"Mack," he said, "I'm here to talk to you about the job you posted. If it's still on the table, I want to put my name in for it."

CHAPTER TWO

JACQUELINE ELLIOT CRINGED as she slammed her employee locker shut. She'd said it was "nice" to spend the night with Everett, as if that wasn't the biggest understatement in history.

Nice! Ha!

In reality, it had been world shifting in more than one way. Her head spun just thinking about it, and she had to swallow another wave of nausea. In fact, figuring out just how world-altering the mind-blowing sex and physical connection had been was part of her after-work plans.

She ignored the three boxes of tests in her bag and thought of that night instead, a night that had come careening back to her the minute she'd laid eyes on Everett in the hall outside his brother's office.

She should have been reticent to go back to his hotel with him, but he'd made her feel so comfortable at the bar with their witty repartee. Not to mention how viscerally her body had reacted to him. Almost instantly she'd felt the flood of heat rush to her core when she'd given him grief about shooting the expensive whiskey and he'd laughed. That sound was still crystal clear in her memory, and she'd done all she could to make him do it over and over.

He'd also backed off when she'd laid out her boundaries not once, but three times at the bar alone. That was sexy as hell, disarming, too.

The first time was when she'd declined his offer to buy her drinks. She didn't need another white knight to come in and save her, someone she'd owe something to afterward. But he'd agreed right away.

The second happened when she'd answered his question about whether she had a partner or not rather abruptly, and he'd merely watched her. She could see the question forming on his lips, but he'd let it go.

Lastly, she'd said she wasn't looking for anything more, not even a friend. She was there to work and concentrate on that and he'd agreed. No pressure, no stress. Just fun.

He'd only partially listened to that, as it turned out, since he had just told her he'd looked for her after they'd gone their separate ways. On one hand, that was incredibly romantic. On the other hand, what did it mean?

Surely the guy wasn't looking for more than a one-night stand, not when he'd told her briefly about traveling for work and not having had a single serious relationship since college.

What it *did* mean, at least she assumed as much, was that he'd felt the same chemistry she had when they'd slept together. Or *not* slept…

Oh, and what delicious not-sleeping it was.

His hands knew just where to touch…his lips where to kiss…the orgasms—plural—had been the most intense of her life. She exhaled a sigh that sounded more like a purr.

Never in her life had she come more than once and even that was a tall order with her ex-husband who considered her to be a vessel for his pleasure and nothing more. That and the angry, at times violent outbursts when she tried to ask for more romance, more love and tenderness, was why she rarely stayed in the same room as him before she'd filed for divorce, citing a headache or some other ailment as her reason for hiding out in the spare room.

That didn't leave much room for sex, certainly not mind-blowing, world-altering sex. Another wave of nausea rocked her like she was a buoy in a storm. It was as if every time she thought of Everett and the amazingness of that night her body reacted like she was allergic to impure thoughts about her one-night stand. Maybe it was more appropriate that she think of him as her nemesis now that she was fighting against him for the job that would keep her in Austin.

The nausea intensified and bile rose up her throat.

She tucked her bag into the locker, procuring one of the boxes of tests. She wouldn't be able to concentrate until she'd put this behind her. There wasn't a real possibility she could be…she refused to say the word.

They'd used a condom the first two times that night. The third he'd pulled out, but she was on birth control.

Still, she couldn't shake the feeling something was wrong. She was two weeks late for her period and her body seemed…off. Like she was walking through a fog with sore breasts and a bloated abdomen.

When she heard voices at the other end of the locker room, Jack tucked the test under her scrubs.

"Did you see that guy? I mean, if more doctors looked like him, people might actually keep their regular checkups."

"No kidding. I heard he's next in line for the trauma doc position. Maybe I won't try so hard to leave Austin after all."

No doubt they were talking about Everett, who'd, of course, already made his mark on the hospital since he arrived yesterday. Why shouldn't he when he'd strolled in with good looks and family connections to the boss.

"I'd let him fix my trauma any day. With those biceps and a bottle of chardonnay, I'd forget Shawn Baylor ever existed." The women giggled.

Jack knew the second voice. It was Tina, a traveling nurse from labor and delivery, someone she'd wanted to get to know more, if only Tina wasn't leaving for her next contract in the Virgin Islands next week. That was the other thing about the temporary assignment Jack had accepted. It left her without the hope of a new support system. Either she'd be leaving in a week's time, or most of the interims would be.

When she'd filed for divorce and fled Boston, she'd left a ten-year career behind. It was safer knowing he wouldn't be waiting outside work in a drunken rage, yelling at her for leaving him and ruining his life, but it was also incredibly lonely starting over alone.

Slamming her locker shut and walking through the room designated for part-time employees made her even more frustrated. She wanted a locker with *her* name on it—her full, maiden name printed and laminated, not written in dry erase each day she took a hospitalist shift.

And up until yesterday, she'd been certain she'd found a way to make that happen. She loved Austin Memorial and the hospitalist work she did there, and so when the job for a longer, more permanent stint had been advertised, she applied and got an interview right away. And she'd been the only candidate, until Everett had come sauntering in.

"You know," she said, coming around the corner, her pregnancy test hidden in her pocket, "being ridiculously handsome doesn't make him the best candidate for the trauma position. Being a good doctor does."

The women, to their credit, nodded and at least had the good sense to acknowledge that they'd been caught gossiping about the physician.

"Yeah, we get it. And it sounds like The Boss is going to give him a trial run at the hospital before offering anyone the job, so he'll get a chance to prove that. Good news for us, since he is, as you pointed out, ridiculously handsome."

They giggled again and gave Jack a wave as they left the locker room. God, would she always feel so out of place? She'd spent so long under Orin's thumb that she didn't get out and meet people who could have become friends. It looked like that wasn't going to happen here, either.

She'd said before that work was the most important thing, and this was further proof why.

All the more reason to take the pregnancy test and get it over with so she could move on and focus on getting this job. Jack's hand trembled so much with the first test, she missed the stick entirely and dropped it in the toilet. She tossed it and started over with the second.

Two minutes later, and she had her answer in the last stall of the part-time employee bathroom. It was a humiliating place to discover she'd broken her rule—no men, only work and rebuilding the life Orin took from her.

Well, that was literally in the toilet now.

The tremble in her hands intensified. How was she supposed to tell the only man she'd slept with in two years that both forms of birth control had failed at their only job? A man who was now standing between her and the job she'd fought for, a job that would give her the clean start she needed. A man she was still, unfortunately, attracted to.

Before she could consider that impossible conversation, though, her pager went off.

Peds trauma. God, anything but that.

It's the job. You signed up for this. And the rest? Well, she'd handle that later, once this crisis was averted. It's not as if the test results were going to change in the next couple of hours.

She cleaned up and ran out the door and didn't stop until she was at the nurses' station.

"What do you have, Trish?" she asked one of the nurses on duty.

"Patient is male, seven years old." Instinctively,

Jack's hand rested on her stomach. *Seven? He was so young...* "MVC on Loop 1. Kid, Riley, was getting something for his mom out of the back seat when they were struck by a wrong way driver. Dad was killed on-site, Mom is in surgery with Mack and you two have the kid."

"Was Riley thrown from the vehicle when it crashed?" Jack was already heading back to the trauma wing.

"Yep. He suffered a head and spine injury at first glance, but we're waiting on imaging. You're on the case with the new guy. He's already in trauma two with the kid doing the workup."

"The new guy?" Of course. Everett Morrison was staying on temporarily to see if he could be a good fit, as was she. Was he starting right away, though? "You mean Dr. Morrison's brother?"

The nurse shrugged. "I guess so. That would explain the same last name and how they both look like they stepped out of the same Gucci advertisement. Anyway, let me know what the scans show. Poor kid."

Jack nodded, then steeled herself for the case. After the results of the test she'd just taken, it was the worst one she could imagine: working on a kid and alongside Everett.

You mean the father of your baby.

That unfortunate thought was the last thing she needed to hear from her subconscious as she ran—literally—into Everett outside trauma room two. She turned the corner and was stopped by a wall of flesh. She stumbled backward, but he caught her. His hands on her skin brought back memories of the night they'd met, the night that led to…

She swallowed back nausea. The night that had led to her situation.

He released her, but not before his scent wrapped around her. It was like being trapped in a pine forest grove, one she wouldn't care if she never found her way out of.

"Hi," he said. Her stomach flipped at the huskiness in his voice. She tried to ignore it, but it was pretty clear she hadn't been in control of her body since she met Everett. Carrying his child wasn't going to help any.

"Hi. I heard we're working together today. Unless you're leaving?"

"No," Everett replied. "I'm not going anywhere." Of course she wouldn't be so lucky. "I wanted you to take the lead on this, so I was actually going to grab his scans for you. I've got him stable for now, but he's been touch and go."

"Why?" Jack asked.

"Well, it looks like he sustained blunt force trauma to his—"

"No. I mean, why do you want me to take lead?"

Everett shrugged and nodded to the room. "You're good with kids, at least that's what my brother said. He's a lot of things, but the best of them is a good judge of character. Was he wrong?"

There had been a moment when they'd been in each other's arms that night a month ago and she'd mentioned family. He'd tensed up and told her he didn't have a relationship with any of them. She hadn't known that included a sibling in the same line of work as him. How much strength had it taken to come ask his brother for a job if they weren't speaking?

"No, I am. Thanks for thinking of me." Or at least, she had been good with kids. Through the window, Jack could see a small body hooked up to a dozen wires and tubes. She'd seen some tough cases in her career specializing in trauma, cases involving children included. But for some reason, this one broke her heart.

He'd wake up to a life vastly different from the one he'd had before the accident. No father, a mother who would hopefully regain her cognitive and physical abilities but need significant PT to recover fully, and his own myriad issues.

"I'll grab those scans and meet you back up here."

She nodded and went in. The beeps and pumps of the machines keeping Riley alive were louder than she recalled them being ever before.

She read through his digital chart and made some adjustments to his meds. Everett came back with the physical scans, and they assessed them together.

"It looks like he'll need surgery to correct two broken clavicles but before that, a ventriculostomy to relieve pressure around his spinal cord," she said.

Everett nodded his agreement.

"Let's wheel him up." They got him upstairs into an operating room for trauma patients and scrubbed in.

While she donned gloves and a gown, Jack watched Everett. She couldn't read the emotions on his face. During the night they'd shared, she'd memorized the way he looked at her when he was driven by lust, how he stared off into the distance when she mentioned family and the furrow of his brow when he talked about how his job might change in the next month.

But this look was new. Was it…fear? Worry?

"Damn. Kid just wanted to help his mom and now his whole life is effed."

"I was just thinking the same thing," she said. It took every ounce of self-control not to feel her stomach, to touch the secret she was hiding. This wasn't the time to tell him. Instead, she grabbed his hand. "You don't have to do this, you know.

You just walked in yesterday looking for a job, and this is a big case to take on."

He shook his head and the creases on his forehead relaxed. "No, I've got it. It's just so different from the kind of trauma I'm used to seeing. At least in racing and the rodeo, the guys choose that life. This isn't at all the same. Riley and his family didn't want this."

She shook her head. She appreciated his honesty, but it highlighted why she was the person for this job, not him. "No, they didn't. Which is why I love what I do. We get to help families piece back together after the worst moments of their lives and hopefully give them some sense of normalcy."

"Hmm," he murmured as they stepped into surgery. "I hadn't thought about it that way. Did you always know you wanted to work with trauma and kids?"

She was grateful for the mask that hid the heat she could feel creeping across her cheeks at the mention of kids.

"Trauma, yes. Kids were more difficult since I knew I wanted to have my own someday. I don't love seeing them hurt or worse on my table, but to some degree, it helps me focus on giving them back to the families that wanted them, you know?"

"I guess. I've never thought about that, about

families wanting their kids and all that. My experience was always a little more…complicated."

"Do you want kids?" she asked. Good grief. Some segue. "I mean, was that ever in your plan? Not to work with, but of your own?"

She was rambling, but thankfully, he didn't seem to notice. They sutured and cut in tandem, and she marveled at how easy it was to work with the man. It was nice, but also a threat to what she was trying to do.

She watched his eyes, the way they glittered under the surgical lights. There was pain there, but also the same focus she had. As they worked, she saw that focus in action and as much as she wanted to find fault in his methods or hate the guy for sweeping in and attempting to steal the job she'd earned, he was good at what he did and a calming presence to work with, too.

Dammit.

"No. Never. My brother, who you know, and I had an unconventional upbringing to say the least. I don't think either of us ever learned how to care for a family thanks to our asshole of a father. Bringing kids into the mix would be—" He shook his head. "It wouldn't be good, let's just leave it at that."

She tensed. *Of course.* She'd left the controlling violence of one man only to end up pregnant by another who wanted nothing to do with kids.

Her luck in picking men was abysmal. It would be comical if it weren't so tragic.

"Got it." They completed the ventriculostomy and clavicle settings. All that was left was to close and wrap up. "Do you have it from here? I've got to finish up with another patient in the ICU."

It was a flimsy excuse, and in the pause between her question and his response, she swore he almost called her out. But in the end, he nodded.

"Yeah. And thanks, Jacqueline." She nodded, ready to leave, to figure out how she was going to hide a pregnancy from a man who wanted nothing to do with the child growing inside her. Anxiety crept over her until he met her gaze. "It was really nice to work with you. I know we didn't meet in the most conventional way and my being here might put us at odds with your goals, but I promise I'll do everything I can to help us both be able to stay."

She opened her mouth to reply, but what could she say? She didn't want another man to tell her he could fix her problems, especially as he gave her three more. Jack was responsible for her own life, her own happiness, and if life had taught her anything?

She could only rely on herself.

"I can handle myself, Everett. Good luck here. It's a good place to work, but if it comes to me or you, I meant what I said earlier—I'm going to fight to stay."

"Of course." She heard the resignation in his voice but chose to ignore it. She didn't actually have a patient to attend to. While it might cost her the job, she needed to come clean to her future boss that she'd be keeping her application for the six-month interim position, but there would be limitations to the kind of medicine she could practice.

If she was going to get—and hopefully keep—this job, she couldn't start off by hiding something so big. Especially since…oh, goodness, she hadn't realized one wild detail.

Especially since my child will be related to my boss. What a nightmare this week was turning out to be.

As she left the room, she stole a glance at Riley lying lifeless on the operating table.

Now, more than ever, Jack was aware of the fragility of life. Medicine had always been her safe place, a slim modicum of control in the chaos of her life. Now, though, she realized how tenuous it all was. One wrong move and she'd lose it all.

The scariest part? What if that move had already been made a month ago, and she was only just now finding out what a colossal mistake it was?

CHAPTER THREE

JACQUELINE HEADED INTO the ER the same time Everett did. She walked with purpose to the nurses' station and picked up her tablet, either ignoring him or not noticing him, he couldn't be sure. He glanced down at his own tablet, trying to look busy while she chatted with the on-call nurses.

She laughed at something one of them said, wiping her hair from her face. Her joy and ease in every area of the hospital astounded him. Everett had been comfortable on a racetrack and in a rodeo arena, largely because none of the eyes were on him. He worked behind the scenes, and if he did his job right, no one knew he existed.

At Austin Memorial, however, people waved at him, smiled and asked him how a particular case went, even went so far as to chat about their cases with him. It was unnerving, being under a microscope like this.

At times he felt the pressure of making precise, right moves like a guillotine above his head. It was crippling.

The only time he didn't feel like he was drowning in a fishbowl? When Jack was around. In part because she drew his focus—with her cascade of brunette waves and deep chocolate eyes that pulled you in, how could she not? But when they were lucky enough to work side by side, she calmed him, almost made him feel as if the rest of the world disappeared.

He could focus better, work longer and ignore the stares of the staff just knowing she was in the same building.

Damn if just her presence wasn't making him a better doctor, and man.

But therein lay the rub. She was growing increasingly distant around him at work, talking to everyone but him, sometimes even failing to meet his gaze. As if to prove a point, Mack sidled up next to her and she smiled at him. She had a different look since he'd met her.

Contentment. She radiated a peace he wished he could cultivate for even an afternoon. It couldn't be because of his brother, could it?

He tamped down the jealousy that rose up his throat like bile.

No, Mack was back with Lainey, his ex-wife, or at least that's how it appeared to Everett. The two talked, flirted and even shared knowing glances across the ER. Everett knew those looks well, since he'd been shooting them at Jack since they'd reunited. Looks she wasn't returning, not since the case with Riley. But every now and then, when she thought he didn't see her, he'd catch her staring, too.

Why couldn't he just ask her what was up?

Because asking is too close to caring, and caring leads to feelings, and feelings lead to... He didn't finish that thought. He liked Jack, sure. Had loved the night they'd spent together and equally loved working alongside her. But that's all he was capable of, so maybe it was a good thing she wasn't meeting his pathological need to get close to her.

That was a prescription he couldn't fill.

Speaking of those, his brother had laid another big—colossal—piece of news on him. He and Lainey were expecting. The two had had infertility problems when they'd been married. That, coupled with the pressures of their jobs pulling them in different directions, had led to them separating and later divorcing. It was kind of nice to see them together again, even if it wasn't "official" or anything.

Still, better Mack than Everett. Now, unwittingly, Mack had met their dad's one request for the men to get their inheritance—procreate. That wasn't ever going to happen to Everett, so thankfully, at least one of the sons was ponying up.

That didn't mean he wasn't interested in getting to know Jack more, though.

"Hey," he said, walking up to his brother and Jack. "I'm consulting on a case from the rodeo if you want to give me a second opinion." It was the lamest excuse he'd come up with yet. Yes, he was doing just that, but this was his specialty, not hers. "She's a thirteen-year-old girl who was barrel racing and got thrown. Just want to go over a treatment plan that gets her back on the horse, literally and figuratively, and could use your peds expertise."

He ignored Mack's quiet stare. If his brother had anything to say about Everett's request, he wasn't saying it then.

"Sure," Jack replied. To Mack, she said, "And sorry, what time did you want to meet?"

"I actually was hoping to catch both of you and speak with you together." Mack's gaze went back and forth between them, as if trying to suss something out.

Not for the first time, Everett wondered if his emotions were on full display any time he was around Jack. If there was a physical manifestation of how his heart rate sped up when she smiled at him, or how his breathing halted in his chest when he watched her tie her hair back before scrubbing into surgery, his feelings would be transparent as hell.

What feelings are those? his asshole subconscious wondered. He didn't have a name, mostly because he couldn't figure out why he was having them in the first place. Why couldn't he have had sex with her and moved on like the rest of his dates? What was this draw to a woman he needed to keep at arm's length?

Not just her—he should keep any woman on the periphery of his life. But Jack especially. She was his competition for a job, she was also crystal clear she didn't want anything more than work, *and* he liked her enough he couldn't risk baring his soul to her and ruining her life in the process. The Morrison men didn't leave relationships unscathed.

Mack patted him on the shoulder as if he had heard every word of Everett's internal monologue and agreed.

"Why don't you two swing by my office in the next half hour before your workup on the girl and we'll iron stuff out."

"Sounds great, Dr. Morrison."

"Can't wait," Everett mumbled. He didn't mind being around his brother as much as he thought he would, but he did wonder what the guy was thinking half the time. They just didn't know each other anymore.

Something in Everett's chest loosened when he was alone with Jack. Forget what he'd said earlier;

he just needed to talk to her, find out why she'd been so distant that week. Then he wouldn't need to make up reasons to work with her so he could be in her vicinity. And maybe then he'd be able to figure out why she got under his skin so much.

"Is the girl already here?" she asked.

"They're on their way. They did an initial workup in the field and wanted to make sure she was safe to transport." He was able to talk about the medical fieldwork without an ounce of regret from pausing that part of his career. Interesting. He thought he'd at least miss it, but the truth was, aside from some of the frustrations related to any kind of career shift, he'd enjoyed his cases. "We can head over any time after lunch once ortho is done triaging."

"Okay, I'm on shift until seven this evening and rounds are done, so just text me when they're ready. But we should go over the rest of the cases that came in last night and then head to your brother's office."

Everett nodded like he wasn't a creepy stalker who hadn't checked her schedule beforehand. Then he realized what she'd said.

"I don't have your phone number." Forget his excuses to see her, to work with her. How lame was not having the phone number of the woman he'd slept with and thought about constantly at work?

"You can page me, too, Dr. Morrison." He tried

not to cringe at the name, but she was keeping him beyond arm's length. Which meant making time to talk to her might be a feat more insurmountable than getting underneath his brother's perfect veneer.

Great. Everett had come to Austin Memorial hopeful he'd, at a minimum, find a job that gave him peace of mind. At best, he'd been excited to reconnect with Mack.

Now, with Mack being mysterious, and adding in Jack's presence, Everett was beginning to think that coming to Austin Memorial was more dangerous than an F1 racetrack.

An hour later, he was sure of it. Mack had them cornered both literally and figuratively. It was one more thing about working in a mainstream hospital Everett hadn't considered—the closed doors, closed windows, closed…everything. In the field, he was outside all day, where even cities boasted fresher air than the hospital.

His skin itched.

"How have things been for you both?" Mack asked.

"Great. It's nice seeing the patients and staff through a different lens than as a hospitalist, even if this isn't necessarily permanent, either." Jack's smile was an affront to everything Everett was feeling.

Everett nodded his agreement, even though, no, it wasn't going as well as she'd made out.

"Yeah, it's fine. How long do you think it'll be till you make a decision?" he asked.

"There are some moving pieces we're still ironing out, so I'm going to ask you two to remain as you are for a couple weeks while we figure them out. Is that okay?"

"Sure," Jack said, her smile still in place. Everett could see the small tic in her jaw that tightened as she said it, though. This was hard on her, too.

"Walk us through what you're thinking," he said to Mack. "Please," he added as an afterthought.

The semantics were simple enough—he and Jacqueline would both continue to be on shift for the next two weeks as an extended interview for the trauma position. That made sense, on paper at least.

But for two reasons, the plan Mack laid out for his work and hire schedule didn't feel right. Partly because it was his brother acting out the role of boss.

It wasn't as if seeing Mack as someone in charge was a stretch. His brother had been serious and managerial since he could drive. When their dad was caught cheating for the umpteenth time, Mack had taken it upon himself to be the man of the family and apparently hadn't stopped, even though he'd moved out at eighteen and never looked back. Even though Everett was a doctor as well, with as much training and experience as his older brother at this point.

So, to have Mack in charge of *him* was another matter altogether.

"Yes, Dr. Morrison, and thank you for the opportunity. I'm looking forward to doing more for Austin Memorial. And thanks for—" Jacqueline glanced quickly at Everett before turning back to his brother "—working with me through my challenges."

Everett watched Mack's face, but as usual, his brother exhibited no emotion other than total control. It was stone cold and emotionless. Had the lion's share of fire and fury just been given to Everett, or was his brother just that much more mature, that much more in control of his own feelings?

"It's my pleasure. Thanks for speaking with me about them, and please let me know what I can do to support you."

She nodded and went to leave. Everett followed her to the door.

"Stick around, Rhett," Mack said. Everett sighed.

It had been two weeks since he'd started work with the trauma team, and this meeting was the closest he'd been to Jacqueline since the first case they'd shared. It was the second part of his discomfort in being trapped in that room—they'd been feet apart and there was still a million miles of distance between them.

Needless to say, watching her walk out without even a glance back at him sucked, plain and simple.

So did his brother staring at him, stoic and silent, the only two adjectives he'd ever used for Mack. At least the guy was consistent.

"Okay, I'm here. What do you need?" Everett asked.

"Are you happy here?"

Everett shot off the first response that came to his head. "Sure. Of course. And I'm grateful for the opportunity."

Mack shook his head. "That's not what I asked. The opportunity has always been there. I told you when you first started that I had a place for you if you wanted it. But this position is a lead into someone I want to hire onto the team full time."

"I know. That's why I applied." Everett didn't know where his brother was going with this line of conversation, but nerves fluttered in his chest, making him feel like he was tachycardic.

Mack nodded. "Okay. So, I'll ask you again. Are you happy here?"

Everett let the question settle between them. Mack, aside from his other endearing qualities, also had a bullshit-ometer that was as finely tuned as his medical skills.

"I'm working on it. This environment is…different. Right now, that's a challenge in some ways, but I'm hoping in time it'll be what I need. A lot of that depends on what happens with the job."

Mack's jaw was tight, his grimace deeper than normal. Not for the first time, Everett wondered if he'd made a mistake in coming here.

"We don't have that kind of time, Rhett. Austin Memorial has two clinics on the east side of town we need to staff in addition to the trauma position here. I need to know who's serious before I commit people to either space."

"Okay, what does that have to do with me? I'm a solid doc with more credentials than almost everyone here, my outcomes are almost always favorable and you know how hard I work when I want something."

The shadow that passed over his brother's face was unmistakable; Everett imagined it each time he spoke to his brother on the phone, when he heard the inevitable sigh on the other end of the line. It was disappointment personified.

"I do. Which is why I wanted to talk to you. As you know, I am only looking at one full-time trauma doc right now, which is between you and Jack." Everett bit his tongue. In any other situation, he'd argue they should be given a fair shot to compete for the position, but this was his brother and Everett had risked everything—his pride and more—to come and ask for help. Now he had to try out? "You may not agree with that, but Jack is the best we've had come through here since I started, and I don't want to lose her."

"And you're fine losing me?" Everett hated that snark was his default mode when he was talking to his brother, but he couldn't help it. Looked like he'd need to start, though, if he wanted to keep this job.

"I'm not fine losing you, but I'm done offering up olive branches where they're not appreciated. So I need you to be honest with me. Are you here to get this position so you don't have to go back to the circuit, or are you here to invest in Austin Memorial and the team?"

"Are you allowed to ask me that?" he asked. "You're the boss."

"As the boss, you're right. I'm not. As your brother, I am. Because there's only one answer that'll land you this job, Rhett, no matter who I am to you. This place has become a working family that chose each other, and I'm asking you to make a choice right now. Either sign up to be part of a team, or let Jack have this job, because she's earned it."

He opened his mouth to add something else, but seemed to think better of it.

That wasn't the first time Everett had heard that about Jack; it's part of why he was so intrigued by her. If the passion he'd witnessed that first night was any indication of how she was in other areas of her life, Austin Memorial would be lucky to have her on their team.

Conversely, if it were anyone but her, he'd put up a fight no matter what his own reasons for being here were; his brother didn't get to dictate that. But because he cared about her to the point of questioning his own motivations, he put aside his ego.

"You gave me a few weeks with her to see how we work together and as part of your preexisting team. Can I use that time to figure out if I fit in as well? If I do, then I promise I'm here to give it an honest try. I can't promise you right now that I can see into the future, that this will be what I need long-term, but I know for a fact that I want to try."

And he did.

Despite the frustrations it came with—Jack's way of confusing his wants and needs, Mack's bossy older brother crap and a confined environment—he still wanted this.

Hell, he *needed* it.

His whole life, he'd been able to flit off to the next gig if he wanted, but now? Sure, he could still do that, but he didn't want to. And that was weird to him. The desire to prove he could be part of a team, part of this team with two people who mattered to him, welled up from some dark place in his chest.

Mack sat on the edge of his desk and crossed his arms over his chest. In that moment, he looked so much like their dad Everett had to swallow back anger that had nothing to do with Mack. Well, not entirely.

"Fine. You can have some time. But I'll be watching how you are with the team, not just your medicine."

"Okay. But, Mack, I'm gonna need a favor from you." Mack eyed him carefully but nodded. Everett was nervous; he'd never stood up to Mack, not really. The closest he'd gotten was living his own life and ignoring requests from Mack that he "come home and settle down."

"Go ahead." God, his brother was born to lead and command, wasn't he? He exuded patience and strength—but Everett knew behind that came pain of his own. It was the only reason he could extend his own patience to his brother.

"I want you to evaluate me the same way you're evaluating Dr. Elliot."

"Obviously, that'll be the case, Rhett—"

Everett shook his head. "No. I know what you mean. Legally, you're going to have the same set of criteria to look at us both for the position. But

I know you'll be thinking about me as a teenager, a young doc right out of med school, even the physician that took the F1 gig a couple years ago. But those men are not who showed up at your door asking for a job. So, if I'm going to be honest with you about what I'm looking for, you need to give me a fighting chance."

Mack's silence was part of his process. Everett imagined him arguing with himself silently before measuring out the perfect response. They were so different, weren't they?

Everett shot from the hip, said what he felt, lived his life out loud. If their dad was going to set them up for failure, at the very least, Everett was gonna live his life without regrets.

"That's fair."

Mack nodded like they were done, and for all intents and purposes, they were. Everett needed to check in with Jack, see if they could work a case together so he could perhaps get a read on why she'd grown so distant from him. When Mack didn't move to walk him out, Everett stopped.

"We done?"

"Have you talked to Dad recently about the inheritance and trust?" Mack asked by way of an answer. Everett was almost stunned silent. This was the one verboten topic between them, largely because it was the one thing they agreed upon. They would do whatever they needed to keep their distance from their old man, which meant their dad wouldn't get a kid out of Everett, and Mack wasn't about to broadcast his new baby news just to earn some money. Their father had tied their hefty inheritance to that one clause: They get someone pregnant and she has the baby, and the boys get their payout. Hell, even their sister had a clause of her own—if she had a baby and used the Morrison name on the birth certificate, she got her payout.

It was so damn archaic it made Everett sick to think about. Enough that he'd usurped his own loneliness to avoid even the possibility of having a baby. He rarely dated, and when he did, it was a night of pleasure—very locked down, protected-from-pregnancy pleasure.

"No, why would he have?"

Mack's silence this time was heavy with meaning. "Just let me know if he does and if you need to talk, okay? I'm saying that last part as your brother, not your boss. Now, wasn't there a patient you and Dr. Elliot were heading to see?"

Everett nodded and left, his steps planted with purpose as he got closer to Jack. Why did he get the sense that his brother's odd conversation was somehow—even loosely—connected to the other conversation he'd overheard between Mack and Jacqueline?

And why did his skin itch wondering how

much more of his life could be upended by family drama? He didn't intend to find out today. No, his brother was right. He had a case to oversee and a beautiful doctor to collaborate with.

That's the only thing he'd let pull his attention from his new goal: Be the best so his brother could finally let go of all the iterations of Everett that had come before, so that he could secure a job that made him feel like he was finally—finally—doing some good in the world.

It was a good feeling he didn't plan on squandering, not even with his dad and that stupid clause lingering in the back of his mind.

CHAPTER FOUR

JACQUELINE SHUDDERED THROUGH a wave of nausea. The smell of antiseptic in the air had always felt safe and like home to her. The hospital was the one place she knew *he* couldn't touch her. But now, around every corner, she was assaulted with visceral reminders that she had messed up again, same as before, by sleeping with a man who had the power to take everything from her.

Even though Everett didn't seem like the kind of man to use his power to control women like her ex-husband, he was still her rival for the one goal she had set her sights on since she'd left the east coast.

A thousand small frustrations plagued her as she tried to distract herself with the case that had come in while she and Everett met with Mack.

The most egregious was the unfortunate realization that the only time she didn't feel ill was around Everett. Something about the citrus and saffron scent that seemed to emanate off him calmed her morning sickness.

Of course. Isn't it just my luck that the one man I need to avoid is the one who makes me feel better?

Yeah, but don't forget he's the same one who created this problem.

Her snarky subconscious wasn't wrong.

"I've seen that look before," a sweet voice said. Lainey Thornton, a fellow doctor on staff, leaned on the nurses' station, biting her bottom lip. The two had shared a couple coffee breaks and some hospital gossip over the past few weeks, and Jacqueline was hopeful it meant, if she stayed, a friendship between the women could blossom. She liked Lainey. "If I didn't know any better, I'd say you were thinking about a specific Morrison brother."

"How…" Jacqueline asked.

Lainey smiled, but there was something reserved about it. "Ugh. I wish I didn't know that unique blend of frustration and lust that came from caring about a Morrison. Do you—" she glanced around, as if to make sure they were alone "—do you have a sec to talk? I could use a friendly bit of advice."

Jacqueline covered Lainey's hand with her own. It trembled beneath hers.

"Of course. Let's move to the locker room?" Lainey nodded and followed her there. The women sat quietly for a bit until Jacqueline broke the silence.

"Lainey, you can trust me if there's something you need to say. I'm a vault."

Lainey's smile fell. "Thanks. I just don't want anything getting back to Everett. Not that you would, but our partners come first, I know that."

"Oh, no. Everett and I aren't—" Jacqueline paused. Did people think she and Everett were together? Oh boy. "Please don't feel you have to share, but if you do, I won't be sharing anything with him. Everett and I…well, let's just say we have a difficult relationship that was made worse by both going after the same job."

"Ha. It sounds like you and I have more in common than I thought. This is about Mack, which is why I worry. He and Everett have such a complicated relationship with their father, who's made this provision that links his sons' inheritance to having a child. Never mind. It's so old-fashioned, and I shouldn't have said anything. Sorry."

Jacqueline prided herself on her composure, bred from a decade of taking hard peds cases and needing to hide her emotions to allow families to express theirs and trust her in kind.

But darn if her jaw didn't drop in surprise. There was so much in Lainey's admission that she needed to process. A pregnancy, potential reconciliation and inheritance? What could she do but nod.

"You and Mack—"

She'd seen Mack and Lainey in some deep conversations, but had never made any assumptions about the root of them. She also hid the fact that she would be directly affected by the pregnancy provision. It had the potential to up end everything, but she couldn't concentrate on that right now. This was about Lainey and Mack.

"Were married. We broke up but lately..." Lainey looked conflicted, and the way she tapped her fingers on the desk said there was so much more to this story. She looked down at her hands. "We've been spending some...time together, if you know what I mean."

Jacqueline nodded. She knew exactly what Lainey meant.

"Do you love him again?"

This time, the grimace was impossible to miss. "I don't know that I ever stopped. But we, well, we went through so much, I just don't know if we can find our way back together." Her pause was heavy, as was the silence filling the space. "The thing is, we have to, in some way. I'm pregnant."

This was big. Like, life-changing big. In so many ways that Jacqueline was still struggling to wrap her head around.

Lainey was pregnant. All Jacqueline could do

was nod like a bobblehead doll, a muted understanding plastered on her face while she patted her friend's the other woman's shoulder. What else could she do? The words stuck in her throat weren't fit for public consumption.

I am, too, she wanted to scream. *I'm pregnant by the other Morrison brother and he doesn't know, and oh, did I mention he doesn't want kids, which is why I haven't told him. But should I know* his *secret? That he'll come into an insane inheritance and won't have to fight for this job if he knew about my...condition?*

"Hmm. That's a lot. I'm here to listen if you need it."

"Thanks. Maybe later I can get you a cup of coffee while we talk through this? It means a lot to have a friend I can go to with this." Lainey smiled.

"I agree. It seems like we have a lot in common, but right now I have to meet my Dr. Morrison on a peds case." Jacqueline caught herself. "Not that he's *my* Dr. Morrison. Just that he's—"

She was spiraling and she knew it. But she was also powerless to stop it.

"I understand. Thanks for chatting. Maybe we can get together tomorrow or this weekend?"

"I'd like that," Jacqueline said, hugging Lainey before they parted ways.

In the span of minutes, her situation had gone

from complicated and scary to FBI cold-case level tangled and terrifying.

Because… Oh, God. Her boss, the one she'd confided her pregnancy in, knew about the inheritance and how it would change his brother's life. Her life. He hadn't said anything, but he had encouraged her to share her condition with the father. It hadn't seemed odd at the time, just a show of support for her to get the help she would need. But now it seemed like…like a warning. She froze in the middle of the hallway.

Does Mack suspect Everett is the father? And if that was the case, what would he do about it? Mack legally couldn't share anything with Everett, could he? No, that was a violation of HIPAA.

But he could make decisions based on what he knew or thought he knew.

The question no longer remained, though. She needed to tell Everett about her pregnancy and let the chips fall where they may. He could tell her again how he didn't want kids, and she wouldn't be any worse off than she was now, imagining how she was going to tackle this pregnancy and fight for a job she wanted—against the father of her child, no less.

At least if he knew, maybe Everett could back off the job now that he wouldn't need this job, specifically. He could practice medicine anywhere.

And she'd be free to work at Austin M. To build a life with her baby safe from the life she'd fled.

It might be boring, a half-life to some people, but that was better than the alternative.

Right?

Then why did her heart lurch when she considered the *other* alternative, one she'd kept far from her thoughts, in case her heart wanted it enough to overlook red flags like she had the first time around.

Love. Which, of course, included companionship. Trust. Partnership.

Passion. Everett's lips on her breasts, on her hips, on her sex came to mind with that last word… His hands roaming and knowing just where to touch to bring her to heights of passion she'd never experienced… Yes, she'd shared that with him, at least.

Yet, she'd mistakenly assumed the rest would follow with Orin. But no, his passion had shifted into something menacing and evil.

Could she…would she risk her future of "good enough" for amazing?

Yes! her heart screamed.

Who was to say Everett would even consider that with her. Raising a child he didn't want and being with a woman he didn't know? Hadn't he also said he didn't date because he couldn't have the commitment?

Ha! Didn't it figure. Jacqueline had allowed herself to become interested in yet another emotionally unavailable man. Lainey might hope to have found love and passion and what seemed like true partnership with Mack, but Everett wasn't Mack. That life wasn't possible for him.

Jacqueline was daydreaming again, all thanks to a good night where she'd been sated physically. When would she learn her lesson? So, where did that leave her? The same place she'd been before.

She took a breath and made her way back to the nurses' station to meet Everett.

When he strode into the ER, he wore a look that she could only describe as steely determination etched on his face. It was so unlike the man she had come to know with a gentle smile and a mischief behind his eyes.

"You ready?" he asked. She bristled. She'd expected the gentle curiosity he'd brought to their interactions the past week, but that wasn't on the table. Had Mack said something to him?

Nerves fluttered in her belly.

"What's wrong?" she asked. Everything in her wanted to keep questions like that to herself. What was going on with Everett was none of her business. But she had something to tell him, and she needed to know his frame of mind before she did.

"Just my brother being…well, the same controlling man he's always been." Nothing about the pregnancy or her.

"Dr. Morrison, Mack I mean, has been fair to me. I'm sorry that's not the case with you." What else could she say? Everett was all passion, all kinetic energy that she couldn't help being attracted to. Where he was liquid fire, Mack was a cool mountain stream, steady and persistent.

Jacqueline got the sense both men could cut through a forest and leave their mark, but not for the first time, she wished she wasn't drawn to the one that could burn her in the process.

"I didn't mean my brother isn't a good boss, but we've had a..." He looked as if he was struggling to come up with the right words. "We've had a rough time getting to a point of understanding one another. Apparently, time and distance didn't smooth that wound."

Jacqueline placed a hand on his forearm, immediately wishing she hadn't. A spark of energy jolted her. Her gaze shot up to meet his, and there it was—the mischief, but this time it was lined with an intensity that was definitely a Morrison trait. He must feel that heat, too, right?

"Um," she said, pulling her hand back, "I just wanted to say family dynamics are complicated, and I'm sorry for any way I've complicated yours."

He took her hand in his and nope—there was

no mistaking the heat between their palms. If he was fire, what would their passion do as a catalyst? They'd burn down everything if they were given the chance.

A thrill whispered across her skin. In a different world, they would be good together. Or have fun at least.

But too much was at stake for her to entertain that now.

"You haven't. I mean, you've complicated my chances at getting this job," he teased. He winked, his playful demeanor peeking through. "But Mack and I are always going to have this dynamic."

"Tell me more about that. You both seem to love what you do, and you're both good at it. Why isn't that enough?" Because if he got his inheritance, at least he wouldn't have to worry about where to find work. He could relocate anywhere.

Everett chewed his bottom lip. She'd pushed, but was it too far? Up until that point she'd avoided Everett at all costs. How else was she supposed to keep a hold on her feelings? And it was imperative she do that—she'd be raising a baby by herself; that much he'd made sure of.

But seeing him with that wounded look on his face made an Everett-sized dent in the armor she'd erected to keep herself safe.

"You'd think so. Let's get into this later, though. Right now, we have a patient to see." The light in his eyes when he spoke about his patients was so magnetic it almost erased the rest of her issues with him. Almost.

"Sure," she said. Although, getting through the day knowing she was keeping a secret from him that would change both their lives was going to be tough. "Tell me about our patient."

Everett launched into the pre-case workup, detailing how young Tanya had been bucked from her horse in the youth barrel racing competition outside town. She'd landed on her spine, but there didn't seem to be any lasting injury to the vertebrae or spinal cord. Inside the room, the young girl looked so much younger than thirteen. She was intubated while the swelling around her brain subsided, and the tubes and wires tracking her vitals and dispensing medicine made the situation appear all the more serious.

According to Everett, it wasn't the last of these injuries they'd see now that spring rodeo competitions were picking up.

Jacqueline took the girl's hand. It was limp and lifeless. Even if she did recover fully, what would that look like for her? Would she be afraid the rest of her life that something might snatch more of her childhood from her?

"I don't know why anyone would take on this kind of risk. And to let a child compete in something so dangerous seems like gross negligence." She shook her head disapprovingly.

"What about playing football? Or hiking in backcountry mountain passes? Rock climbing? Scuba diving? They're all dangerous. Where do we draw the line?" Everett asked. The edge to his voice said this was personal to him.

She understood what he was saying; it was the same argument most parents of her patients made. "I get it. And your point is a valid one, but don't you think there's enough risk out there in the world without purposely creating it, and for what? A quick jolt of adrenaline?"

This was personal to her, too. Her parents had been gamblers, leaving them destitute and poor until Jacqueline was old enough to leave home and make sure she never took that kind of risk again. Then, of course, she'd fallen in love—or what she'd thought was something close—with Orin. The physical risk he put her in made her realize she'd never be okay with jeopardizing her safety and health. Not for any reason.

Everett's stare was unrelenting. "Jack—" he started. "Sorry, Jacqueline. I'm sorry for whatever happened to you that made you feel this way, but feeling alive for a moment is sometimes the only way these kids, or adults, will find out what they're made of."

"And there aren't other ways of finding that

out? Without this as a possibility?" She pointed to the lifeless body on the hospital bed being kept alive by machines.

"This," Everett said, "is possible no matter what. She could have been hit by a car outside her house, or tripped coming down the stairs. Risk is everywhere, Jacqueline, and our job isn't to mitigate it, but to make sure families get the chance to keep making amazing memories with their loved ones. And to your other question? I'd rather feel alive for one day and have those I love feel that way than live a lifetime of playing it safe and never knowing true joy or adventure."

Jacqueline felt heat behind her eyes. Darn her surging hormones. It wasn't that what Everett was saying was particularly different from what she believed; he just saw "living a life of adventure" differently than she did.

"Yeah, I guess."

"Listen, she'll be okay." Everett held Jacqueline's gaze. It was penetrating and honest, but lacked in judgment. "She's been triaged by ortho and once the swelling goes down, they think she'll recover with the right treatment plan. That's where we come in. But, if this is too difficult for you, I'll understand if you want to bow out."

She shook her head. She was a physician; taking the Hippocratic oath meant not only doing no harm, but helping wherever she was able. That did not include deciding whether a patient deserved care or not.

"Of course not. I'm here to help Tanya in any way I can. But putting aside our clear difference of opinion on the seriousness of participating in these sports, you and I are trauma docs. We don't make long-term treatment plans for patients. That's the physical therapist's job."

Everett nodded as he stood at Tanya's bedside, checking the chart against his own workup.

"You're not wrong. But they're asking me to consult since I've got so much experience with rodeo injuries. I've worked ten years jumping back and forth between that circuit and the F1 racing one, and there aren't many injuries I haven't treated."

"I didn't know you dedicated so much of your time to that field of medicine." What he must've seen during that time.

"Yep. Most of my career." There was that shadow across his face again. Was this where he and Mack butted heads? Jacqueline had only worked for the older Morrison brother for a little over a month, and she already knew he was measured, steady and avoided everything resembling risk. It wasn't a stretch to imagine they might disagree about how to live their lives and careers.

"I'm glad those athletes had someone like you to help them." She meant that. It took a special person to put themselves in dangerous situations to help others. Even if Everett wasn't ever in immediate danger himself, he'd lived a life of rootlessness to make sure people chasing their dreams could be safe doing so. There was honor in that, and her armor cracked just a bit more.

"Um, thanks. It needed to be done and I enjoyed that life, until I didn't."

What was the story there? And why did Jacqueline feel an overwhelming desire to know it, along with everything else about the man?

She blamed the life growing inside her, a life that connected Everett to her in a visceral, permanent way. Every time she remembered that, a wave of nausea threatened to crash over her, but she kept it at bay. Fighting those moments was going to be as difficult as finding the right time to tell Everett what she needed to.

Maybe when they were done here, she'd pull him aside. One thing was certain. He needed to know so he could make some decisions of his own.

Everett made some notes on Tanya's chart and handed them over to Jacqueline to see.

"I like this," she admitted. He was a brilliant doctor, that much was obvious. She agreed with his assessment. They'd wait till the swelling subsided and Tanya was out of the woods there, then they'd work on her PT not to regain basic range of motion, but to build back strength in some of the areas she'd atrophy in healing her more serious injuries.

Everett was thorough and efficient, his work without reproach.

"Can I ask why you chose it? This kind of work, I mean."

"Do you mean what we're doing here at Austin Memorial, or what I did with the racing and rodeo teams?"

"That last one." Though she was curious about the shift he'd made and the timing of it. "But later, I reserve the right to add in why you came to Austin Memorial." She winked and tucked the laugh he responded with inside her heart for later. It was such a sweet sound, and she found it grounded her, made her happy to hear.

Interesting.

"Sounds good. Well, it's kind of a long story, but the short version is I never wanted to settle in one place too long. My dad left us a pretty unconventional life blueprint, and moving with a job was my answer to that."

"Did he move around, too?"

"Yes, we did," Everett said, his smile vanishing. There was a story there. "But each place we moved, he put on a front of a big, happy family and then hid a whole life of infidelity and cheating business from us. Mack and I swore we'd never be like him and just chose opposite ways of manifesting that, I guess."

He tried to laugh it off, but she could hear the pain in his voice.

"Anyway, I didn't want to live anything but my authentic life out in the open, and since rodeo and racing isn't for me as much as medicine, I figured I could at least travel with the teams and help where I was needed."

"I admire you," she admitted. It felt silly to say, but it was true. "I've never had the courage to live out loud. This job is the closest I've come to it."

"I'd like to know more about that, Jacqueline," he said. He was close enough to touch, for his scent to wrap around her good sense and choke it.

"Call me Jack." His smile was so immediate, so effervescent, she came undone. So much for making smart choices where Everett Morrison was concerned.

"Well, we're done here, Jack" he said, clearing his throat. "I've got another case, but afterward, can I buy you a cup of coffee?"

"I'd like that." Neither of them moved toward the door. If anything, some force of nature or magic seemed to have moved them closer to one another.

She shook her head, breaking the fog being this close to him put her in. "Actually, before you leave, can I talk to you for a minute?" she asked. "It's important."

She needed to get this out now, while she still had the courage. Something about this time with Everett, the most she'd spent in his presence since they'd cared for Riley, was unraveling her plans.

"Of course. Whatever you need, Jacqueline. I know you think of me as your rival, but I'm… I'm not. I want to be here for you, too."

His earnest answer calmed her racing heart. There wasn't ever any hesitation with him, but would that all change in a moment when she shared her secret? There was only one way to find out.

"Do we need privacy?" he asked. Thank goodness his brain was working enough to think about that.

She nodded. "Yes, please."

He ushered them out of Tanya's room and opened an on-call room, motioning for her to step inside. Before she could open her mouth and let her secret spill, however, their pagers went off just as a Code Blue was called over the speakers.

Jacqueline's heart thumped loud in her chest as she glanced down at her pager. Her gaze shot up to meet Everett's.

"Tanya," they said in unison and tore off toward the young girl's room, Jacqueline's secret tucked tightly back in her chest for safekeeping.

Please let us be in time, Jacqueline thought. *Please let this little girl be okay.*

CHAPTER FIVE

EVERETT WORKED QUICKLY. His hands flew over the cords and tubes that could be disconnected, tearing them from Tanya's young, frail body. Jack did the same, seeming to mirror his work without getting in his way. She was intuitive, intelligent and calm even as she hurried to get the girl prepped for emergency surgery.

"Can you—" he started.

"I already called ahead and let them know we'd be headed down and to have the neuro operating room ready to go."

"Perfect, thanks." He added "efficient" to the list of adjectives he'd use to describe Jack if he were the one evaluating her for the job. For so many reasons, it was a good thing he wasn't.

You think it's better to be going against her? When the other words that come to mind when you think of her are "magnetic, passionate, alluring"?

He ignored his overactive brain and concentrated on the crucible that was the hallway system at Austin M on a weekend. It was heinous and congested with patients and staff, reminding Everett of the racetrack in the middle of a circuit.

They arrived at the operating room and within minutes were scrubbed in and ready to relieve the swelling in Tanya's brain that was causing her to crash.

Jack stepped in to his left, assuming the assisting position.

"No," he said. "Take the lead."

"But she's your consult," she said.

"She was while we were coming up with a way to get her back in a saddle. Right now, you're the expert, Jack. Tell me what you need."

As if the world itself shifted, Jack's lips pressed in a knowing smile and her confidence radiated. If he'd been impressed by her before, it was nothing compared to when she took the helm in the operating room.

"We're prepped for a craniectomy, but she'll have better outcomes with a ventriculostomy."

He didn't disagree. He instructed the nurses and anesthesiologist to get Jack what she needed for the less invasive procedure. Her shoulders were thrown back, her eyes focused above her mask. She was a vision to watch at work, that much was certain.

"I need the drill and tube ready to go. When I

say, I'm going to need you to take the equipment so I can place the drain."

"You've got it. How would you like me to assist?"

Jack instructed him through her version of this procedure, the same as for an adult, with some minor adaptations given Tanya's small body. Each hole she bored, each cut she made was precise and methodic.

When Tanya's blood pressure spiked, Jack didn't flinch. She simply found the third bleed in Tanya's brain, released the pressure and kept at the surgery until all the patient's vitals were back in a healthy margin.

Everett glanced up and exhaled when they were sure they were out of the woods. In the gallery window, Mack stood over them, his arms crossed tight over his chest. Per usual, his brother's face belied no emotion, leaving Everett guessing for the umpteenth time what he could be thinking. Before he could wonder aloud, Mack was gone.

Hmm. Was that observation part of the assessment? Surely it was, but it could go either way. On one hand, Everett had deferred to a colleague for the surgery, showing he was a team player. On the other hand, it was Jack who'd shone in the moment, Everett just a side character in her show.

Not that he'd have had it any other way. Watching her was awe-inspiring. He'd met good docs in his line of work before coming to Austin Memorial. But he could always pinpoint those who were good at their jobs because it was part of the gig and they had studied and practiced, and those doctors who had done all of the above and also loved what they did. Watching those doctors, docs like Jack, was like watching a finely choreographed dance.

"It was a pleasure working with you, Jack," he said as they closed and prepped the patient to be moved to the peds ICU. "You're incredible in the OR. Have you seen the new trauma site? Mack said it would have a peds wing, and I can't imagine anyone else would be a good fit for running it."

He caught a hint of blush above her mask. Humility looked as alluring on her as her curves, her wavy hair draped over a shoulder when she wasn't in surgery… As the rest of her.

"Thank you. And, um, now that Tanya is out of the woods, can we have that conversation?"

He nodded, nerves accelerating his already racing heart.

After the way they'd connected that first night together, he'd thought she felt something more for him as well. But they'd agreed on one night, so they'd gone their separate ways. Then he'd run into her on his first day at Austin Memorial and he'd gotten the sense that she'd missed him, too.

Until they'd shared Riley's case.

They'd been talking, joking even, as they worked in perfect synchronicity. Then he'd answered one of her questions—was it about kids? Or families? He couldn't recall the specifics now. Only that she'd grown distant and she hadn't reached out to him since.

Until today.

Here's the thing: He shouldn't care. He was there to work and to try something different because the world of medicine in F1 racing and rodeos was exhausting and breaking him down. This was his pause button to assess what he wanted next, and he knew with absolute certainty what he didn't want—a relationship that would lead to nothing but heartache.

Between his biological predisposition to run when things got tough, the way his father reinforced that through his own behavior, and his own troubled past with being left behind, what hope did he have in love?

None. Which was why it confused the shit out of him that he wanted Jack. Like, deep in the pit of his chest where only his secret longings took root. He watched her work and connect with patients, heard her laugh across the hospital lobby, and he wanted more of both. More of her.

After over a month of radio silence from the woman, now she wanted to talk to him. The "why" of it itched at a part of his brain he should listen to more, but then he gazed down into those liquid chocolate eyes and was lost to anything other than following her into the on-call room behind the nurses' station.

He didn't care who saw them, didn't care if word got back to his brother. He only wanted to follow Jack wherever she went and hell bring him the consequences later.

When the door was shut behind them, Jack whispered, "I'm pregnant." But he'd heard that wrong, he had to have. Because she spoke so quietly and faced away from him, he'd misunderstood what she was telling him.

"I'm sorry, you're going to have to repeat that, because—" he laughed, the sound inappropriate and loud in the quiet room "—you're gonna love this. It sounded like you said you're pregnant."

He chuckled, his head shaking at the absurdity of that. Imagine if that were true. That would mean he'd be inextricably tied to a woman who he was in direct opposition to. Then—and this was the silly part that brought on another round of anxious laughter—his father would have gotten exactly what he wanted from both of his sons. The irony, when the brothers had done everything they could to keep their old man from stepping over the boundaries they'd laid for him.

An heir—two, in fact—and proof that the Morrisons were virile men sowing their seed all over kingdom come. It was enough to turn his stomach.

Jack turned to face him, her smile nowhere to be seen, and damp eyes replacing the giant, inquisitive orbs from before.

"So that we're both perfectly clear, that's exactly what I said, Everett. I'm pregnant. And, before you collapse into another fit of giggles, it's yours. I haven't been with anyone but you since I left my husband years ago."

Everett felt behind him, found something solid to latch on to—a desk chair by the feel of it—and collapsed into it.

"We're pregnant," he said, putting his head in his hands. It was stuffy in the room, and drawing a breath was getting more and more difficult. He sat up and breathed deep, but it didn't do anything to make him feel as if he wasn't dying of an arrythmia.

"Yes. Technically, I am the pregnant one, though. I never understood couples who said 'we' when they talked about pregnancy as if the man had to give up shellfish and red wine. Like he had to trade green tea for his espresso, walking for his long runs, and sparkling water for wine at night."

"Couples? Are we—" he started, and then the breathing thing got worse.

"No, before you go tachycardic and we have to

get a crash cart in here, I'm not making any assumptions we're together. That would be pretty irresponsible, wouldn't it? When we're not both going to be hired? No, I just wanted you to know so we could talk about what comes next."

When he'd come into the room, he'd been prepared for doing anything needed to get the woman just feet from him to talk to him, to go out to dinner and find out more about her. He'd craved being a part of her world, even for a little while.

Never, in his wildest imagination, however, did he think about being part of her world for the next two decades while they worked through raising a child together. That was, if she chose to—

"Are you keeping it?" he asked. Fearing that the next breath would drag him under its depths, he held it. Hearing her answer was more important than anything, oxygen included.

"I want to. But that shouldn't mean anything for you. I don't need you to be involved or to pay for anything. I just..." She touched a hand to her belly and he winced. "I can't imagine a life without this little human in it now that they exist."

He agreed. God, despite the heaviness of this news, despite the ways it changed everything, it was a miracle he couldn't imagine not having. He tried to say as much but the words stuck in his throat as if he'd been intubated.

He was blowing it. Asking all the wrong things,

keeping too much distance between him and Jack and… And the baby they'd made together. He was going to be a dad, which on the flip side of the miracle part of things, meant that despite everything Everett had done to prevent this exact scenario, his father had gotten what he wanted.

"Does my brother know?" he asked. It was an asshole question; he knew it the second it was out of his mouth. But the last thing he needed was another "I told you so" from a guy who had at least a dozen more of those up his sleeve.

"No, I told my *boss* that I was pregnant, and he was professional enough not to need to know the sordid details. But good to know you've got your priorities straight."

He closed his eyes. He deserved that.

"I'm sorry, I'm just processing this, along with a hundred other things. Give me a second, please. I'm not gonna get this right on the first try."

She opened her mouth, but whatever she'd been about to say was silenced by their pagers going off.

"Jacqueline, can we talk about this? Please?"

"We just did."

She gathered her things, her cheeks red, her mouth pulled tight in what looked like disappointment. He didn't blame her; he'd handled her news as poorly as he could have.

"Wait. I want to talk when we're done and I've

had some time to think about all the ways this impacts me—and us, of course. Can we do that?"

"The ways this impacts *you*?" God, he couldn't say, couldn't do anything right, could he? But the news had been life changing. He was still reeling from the five words that had altered everything. *I'm pregnant...and it's yours.*

"I just meant that this is a big deal for me, too."

"Ha!" she said. "Please tell me more, Everett. You're the brother of the guy in charge of hiring here, and your stomach and life aren't going to be completely changed if you choose to ignore this. Meanwhile, I've fought to even get here." She wasn't wrong, but still, it's not like he was going to actually ignore this. He could, though, and his life wouldn't change a bit. Except he'd know that out there, somewhere, was his flesh and blood. It would be unconscionable to pretend otherwise, and biologically, he knew it would be impossible. "Do you know who and what I've fought?"

Before he could nod, she lifted her scrub shirt and pointed at the burn scar along her abdomen.

"I fought my husband off me after he poured burning wax on my chest and stomach. He said I deserved it because I set out candles, hoping to help him see how much I wanted time alone together, that I wanted him. But he was tired, and I was 'always working at the hospital,' where he thought I was sleeping with another doctor. He thought the candles were an act of guilt instead of what they were—an olive branch to connect us again. This is one of a dozen stories like that. So, I left. I made a life for myself, and the only time I've broken my own rule—to not let a man close enough to see these scars, or to get in the way of what I'm trying to rebuild, or to have control over my decisions—was with you. And look at what happened. I ended up pregnant, which means I broke all three rules. Good grief. I'm like an after school special of what not to do. But sure, let's talk more later about how this might impact you getting a job working for your older brother."

Everett ignored the accusation of nepotism. The reality was there—he had the upper hand when it came to the job and he would be a royal ass if he denied it. But none of that mattered in light of everything else she'd just shared. He'd seen his fair share of scars inflicted by life and circumstance. He'd also seen the scar on Jacqueline's stomach when they'd made love and attributed it to a childhood injury. If he'd have known what *really* caused it, he'd…

He'd what? Go find the guy and rough him up for hurting a woman? He was a doctor who'd taken a vow never to harm another. But the rage inside him boiled and didn't seem to realize that.

"Where is he?" Everett growled. The trill and beep of machines in neighboring hospital rooms punctuated the silence while he waited for her reply.

"Why does it matter to you? Are you planning on fixing this for me? Because you can't."

"No," Everett said. "But I want to make sure he can't hurt you ever again. Jack—"

"Careful," she said. "We may be tied by the… situation I find myself in, but we're still rivals at work. It's Dr. Elliot or Jacqueline going forward. I'm sorry I blurred the lines, but it won't happen again."

"Jacqueline," he said, refusing to believe they were only rivals. They'd made a *child* together, and even though he hadn't known that at the time, he knew he wanted to be around her more, even the day after she'd left his bed. It wasn't the baby that connected them, it was something else, something more. "This guy sounds dangerous. I'm not trying to be your friend or anything else, but you have to let me know if you're safe. You're carrying my—our—child."

"He's not here and he'll never find me. What matters is that I take care of myself and my baby and that means doing the best job I can here. You can help me by allowing me to work. The rest I'll figure out on my own, like I've done for everything else in my life."

"Jack, please." He reached for her, but she evaded his touch, her eyes lined with moisture.

"Don't. Call. Me. That. We're not friends; you made sure of that."

Shit. His chest ached with need—to go to her, to take her in his arms and hold her while they figured this out, to run away with her and never look back on his past and all the complications it made for his future.

He let her leave, knowing he'd see her again in a couple minutes either way.

Alone with his thoughts, they pelted his brain, making it a long walk to the ER.

She's been hurt by someone she cared for, maybe even loved.

She's pregnant. It's your baby.

You're going to be a father. Going to have a child with another person, someone who has been hurt—physically and otherwise. Both of them will need you to show the hell up. They'll need to count on you.

He could do that. Hadn't he always come through when he'd been needed? Even if a particular decision wasn't his first choice, he'd somehow found a way to make things happen that needed to. Take the death of his and Mack's mom, for example. He'd put on a brave face, been the son he needed to be while they buried her, then let his brother dictate how and when they were allowed to grieve. All he'd wanted to do was collapse, followed by coming to blows with their father for running her down emotionally to the point that she gave up when she got sick.

One more thought sat at the periphery of his consciousness, and now that it was close enough to touch, it burned.

You've earned your inheritance, at least.

Does Jack know about the trust? It was an intrusive thought, one that he needed to ignore if he was supposed to concentrate on work the rest of the day—or ever again.

But then it spiraled into its darkest iteration.

How long has she known she was pregnant? If she knows about the trust, is that the only reason she told me about the baby? Because she expects a payout?

It didn't make sense with what he knew about Jack. She wasn't the type of person who would use another as a way to get ahead; that much he was certain about. But the doubt had planted itself, become a malignant cancer that ate away anything healthy.

Talk to Mack and see what he told her.

Then a memory surfaced, a recent one from their meeting earlier. Mack had asked him if he had heard from their dad about the trust. The timing of that seemingly innocuous question couldn't be circumstantial, could it?

Everett strode into the ER, desperate for the case that he'd been paged about. He needed a distraction, and once again was frustrated by the confines of the hospital. At least at the rodeo arena or racetracks there was danger lurking around every corner, giving him something to distract himself. Here, all he had was a pervasive fear he'd run into Jack or his brother before he got a handle on how he felt. It was suffocating.

As were the implications of this. If it was only him and Jack who had to find a way to work together to make a plan, it was fine. They worked well together, and he had a suspicion that translated outside of work as well. But it wasn't that simple.

Mack was observing them to see who he wanted to hire. Ostensibly, Everett had a leg up—physically at least. He knew the limitations of a pregnant woman and how much she could lift, how long she could stay on her feet. But he didn't want the job because he'd gotten Jack into her… situation.

Then there was the other part of his reality. If he didn't want to, he wouldn't have to work again. The golden parachute his father guaranteed meant his sons would want for nothing if they granted him a single thing—another Morrison to carry on the name.

Despite his objections, he'd made that come true, but that didn't mean he had to accept his father's bribe. He might have gotten a woman pregnant, but he could still forge his own way in life.

Forget his brother knowing if he was the man responsible for Jack's condition. He couldn't let their dad know he'd somehow, some way, gotten exactly what he'd wanted.

Which meant one thing: He needed to have another awkward conversation with Jack to find out what she knew. Then, he'd make a plan to ensure that she and his child were taken care of, and that meant keeping them as far from Thom Morrison as possible.

CHAPTER SIX

JACK WALKED THE hill off Sixth Street, marveling at how warm the air was, despite only being the end of March. She was winded at the top, something she'd have to get used to as the tiny being growing inside her took more and more of her body's resources.

It was such a miracle being pregnant, a biological phenomenon she'd been curious about even beyond the medical applications. But going through it herself added a layer of pride and wonder that she'd never had when she cared for pregnant women. Back then, she'd held a natural curiosity with perhaps a mild jealousy at women who were lucky enough to have a baby and start a family with those they loved.

The jealousy remained, but she pushed it aside in a reality check. She wasn't having a child with a partner, and sure, she'd be taking on this adventure alone with no family support, but she was having a baby. Wasn't that enough? The rest would come—or it wouldn't—but she'd made a new member of a family and would always have that, at least.

She checked her pulse since it felt a little fast. There was so much she'd had to get used to the past few weeks as she adjusted to her new reality. The urge to pee just minutes after drinking a glass of water, for one. Then there were the myriad changes to her diet. She'd already had a relatively healthy relationship with food, but now she was held to strict standards that Mel, one of the OBs in the new birthing center they'd acquired, had given her to follow. She wasn't the only one, either.

The growing life inside Jack was picky. She—or he, she admitted, though her finely tuned intuition told her she was going to have a little girl—wanted small portions of food, only half of what Jack was used to consuming during meals. But she wanted double the quantity of mealtimes, so Jack had to carry snacks with her everywhere she went. On her rare days off, like today, she felt uniquely split between eating and using the restroom.

Soon, those challenges would be following her to work. Jack put her hands on her head in a sorry attempt to open her lungs and catch her breath, but it did nothing. How was she supposed to do her best work to get this job if she was so tied to her own physical changes?

She bent over, stretching her tight hamstrings. *I need to get out and enjoy the city more.* The sun was setting over Lady Bird Lake, which was really a nicer name the locals had given to the Colorado River. Bats from the bridge over the river dove in the waning light, picking insects for their meals midflight.

Leaning to one side, she bounced, feeling the flex in her tired muscles. She'd barely gotten over her morning sickness that afternoon and now felt it creeping back. Why they attributed it to a time of day when the feeling could roll over her at any time was a medical misnomer she vowed not to repeat with her patients if she was lucky enough to get the job.

"Hey, there, Jack. I mean, Jacqueline."

The smooth-as-whiskey voice warmed her skin as much as it gave her chills up her spine.

Jack's gaze shot up, and the blood formerly in her head fled south and pooled in her lower abdomen. She also lost her balance at the surprise interruption and almost fell. A solid mass of flesh stopped her from toppling to the ground, however. She was careful not to move too quickly and have yet another wave of nausea bowl her over—another expected but unfortunate side effect of her pregnancy.

"Everett," she said, steading herself. "Hi." The rest of the words she'd planned on snapping back with—that she could walk wherever she chose, for starters—died on her tongue when she caught a glimpse of him. He wore a pale-blue button-down chambray shirt with snug jeans and a pair of cowboy boots that were the only part of his outfit that looked worn. The shirt brought out the color of his eyes, and with him standing in the forefront of what was turning out to be one of the top ten sunsets of her life, the embarrassment hit.

She'd been caught ass up in the air by a man she was horribly attracted to, a man she'd also carefully avoided outside work obligations for the past few weeks. A man she'd given the riot act to, and only recently had realized how unfair she'd been. But what could she say that would fix things? What was there to fix, even? They were having a child together, but neither could be in a relationship, so maybe it was better to let things lie where they were. At worst, it was a buffer between her feelings for the man and her knowledge that they were wildly inappropriate.

Except, said man was there, invading her fragile peace, and looking like sin on a cracker while doing it.

Great.

"You look—" he started. Thankfully, he didn't finish that sentence before she was forced to whack him with her fanny pack for pointing out that she was disheveled, yes, but it wasn't as if she was heading out to dinner on Rainey Street or to work. She was on a walk, for crying out loud. "Anyway, it's really good to see you. I feel like we've been missing each other at the hospital lately. I didn't expect to find you on this side of town."

"I live over here," she replied. She didn't dare mention why they'd been missing one another at the hospital. She'd been doing her level best to ignore and avoid the man, lest she'd have to explain her reaction—poor, at best—to how he'd handled the news that she was pregnant with his baby.

"You drive all the way to the east side of town to work?" he asked.

She frowned. "No. I take the bus all the way to the other side of town. An apartment was my first priority when I left, but it's fine. A car is a necessity only if I'm leaving the city, which I'm not."

The look on Everett's face was unreadable. When she'd first started as a temporary trauma doctor at Austin Memorial, she'd been told that Mack was the hardest man to read, with his stoic, lingering gazes as he assessed doctors and programs and worked with tough cases.

But by a long shot, Jack found Everett to be the more unreadable of the two Morrison brothers. His brows were always pulled up in curiosity, but he rarely explained what he was thinking, leaving an air of mystery.

"I can pick you up, you know. I live just at the bottom of the hill." The temptation was strong to accept, if only it wasn't an opening of sorts, a softening to the hard line she needed to draw in the sand between them; it was hard enough to keep that line intact carrying the man's baby and working alongside him as he actively saved lives in front of her. If she wasn't careful, she'd trip over the line and fall head over heels for the guy. Especially if he kept being so nice to her when she really didn't deserve it.

On the other hand, she'd almost been late to a work shift on two separate occasions thanks to a delay in the public transportation schedule. "You don't have to answer now, but Jacqueline, I want to help you in any way I can. I mean that. I know I was an ass when you first told me, but I had a lot to process."

She held up a hand to stop him. "No. You reacted the way I would have if I didn't have any warning my life was about to irrevocably change. I'm—" She inhaled, lowering her fortification just a little. What could it hurt? "I'm sorry. I should have given you time to process."

He chuckled. "I've had the time, but now I'd like to talk about it with you, if it's okay? Do you have plans right now?"

She fought the urge to tell him that yes, she was heading home, then on a date or something that he couldn't fight. But this was the father of her child. She owed him time so they could figure this out together.

"I need to shower, but then, yeah. I have some time. Where do you want to meet?"

His lips twisted in thought. It was adorable, the way he worried his bottom lip between his teeth when he was thinking. She noticed he did that when he read patient charts, too.

"Let me pick you up and we can come back to my place. I have a fully stocked kitchen and wouldn't mind making you some dinner to make up for my poor behavior earlier this week. Rice and grilled chicken with peppers sound okay?"

Her stomach betrayed her by rumbling loudly at that precise moment. She grimaced. "Sure. What can I bring?"

"Nothing. This will give me a chance to impress you with my culinary prowess," he said, winking at her.

As if she needed one more thing to be impressed with when it came to Everett Morrison.

"Send me your address and I'll pick you up in a half hour. Is that enough time?"

Jack nodded, avoiding a glance at her outfit, knowing her hair was in a pile atop her head in two thousand knots. She would need a year and whole beauty department to feel herself. Two years to feel beautiful enough to be in a private space with Everett-the-dreamy-doctor. Everett-the-father-of-her-baby.

Half an hour later—and four flights of stairs that were becoming increasingly harder to manage each day of her pregnancy—and she'd put on the most "date-ready" outfit she owned and didn't feel any better than she had in sweaty tights.

When she opened the door to her apartment, Everett was there in black slacks and a white polo. His gaze traveled over her and as if his hands had done the same thing, she felt a touch in each part of her body that he looked at.

"Wow. You look—" He cut himself off again and she knew it. She was bloated, and her skin was greasy from the hormone shifts her body endured as it grew her tiny human. "You look amazing. I mean, it was one thing to be amazed seeing you active and outside the hospital, but this is... well, you're gorgeous."

She'd have accused him of overselling or pandering if it weren't for the awe in his eyes. When he handed over a granola bar, she could have kissed him. She'd meant to eat right after her walk, but getting ready for her...whatever this was, took the whole time.

"Also, someone left this in your door." He handed her a letter.

"Thanks, Everett." She perused the letter and devoured the granola bar, her propriety be damned. Forget flowers, candy, cards… This man knew just what she needed, and there was something totally sexy about that. If there was any reason anything should be sexy about the man she was supposed to be avoiding, that was.

"What's it say?" he asked, when she frowned. The man was in tune with her moods, that was for certain.

"It's a letter reminding me that my interim stay is almost up. I didn't sign a permanent lease because, well—"

"You don't have a permanent position," he said. She nodded, ignoring the heat building behind her eyes. If just one thing could go her way…

"Anyway," she said, shaking her head and trying on a smile, "shall we?"

They drove to his place, the whole time Everett sneaking glances at her. If she didn't know any better, she'd think this was a date.

But that couldn't be right. Because Everett wasn't looking to date any more than she was. Especially now.

One intrusive thought lingered in the back of her mind. The trust fund. She'd yet to speak to him about that, and whether he'd consider using it to buy himself time to seek out other places to practice and letting her have the job.

You want him to leave? her inner critic chimed in. No, she didn't. Not anymore. But Everett staying put him in opposition to her other goals—namely to have a place to work and feel safe.

Even though this wasn't a date, it felt wrong to bring all of this up at that moment.

Still, when was a good time? They were nearing the end of their observation period, and Mack would be making his decision soon.

Jack gasped when they got inside Rhett's apartment. He might've had a few sweet words to say about her outfit, but it was downright simplistic compared to the vaulted ceilings, walnut floor-to-ceiling bookshelves, and oh—the view of the Austin skyline. The sun had set, but there was a gradient from a deep orange to a midnight blue. In the center of the scape was their four-story hospital, lit up from within.

"Everett, this is stunning. How did you score something so nice this close to downtown in peak season?"

Everett shrugged. "Some of my F1 clients keep places in the cities they race in and loan them out when they're not in town. I've got it until the US Grand Prix comes back to the Circuit of the Americas next year."

Jack sighed. It was so beautiful, this view of the lake, of the city… She'd been happy to have a place with laundry in the apartment, regardless of its flights of stairs and impermanence, and meanwhile this man whose luck knew no boundaries was blessed with a spectacular view and barely had to pay a cent.

It wasn't fair, but then, what was? The man was also sitting on a golden payout that would set him up for life, or at least afford him the chance to make a life anywhere, and had the audacity to turn his nose up at it so he could live life on "his terms."

She understood the compulsion to buck a family life that wasn't healthy, and the bravery it must take to walk away from that kind of life-changing money, but when he had the kind of financial security he did, it sure made choices like that infinitely easier to make.

"This view makes my heart hurt. I think I'd lose my job simply for the opportunity to watch the sun rise over the water."

"Here, take a look at this." He'd opened his phone and pulled up a photo.

"My God. This is breathtaking. Did you take this here?"

He nodded, a soft smile on his face. Why did he have to be so gosh darn seductive when he made simple gestures? Or was part of his seductiveness the way his arm was casually draped on the couch behind her, his citrus scent clinging to her libido, reminding her she'd made a child with this man?

"I did. Check out the past week. I take a photo each morning before I come in, but I'm not sure what I'll do with them. I think I just feel lucky enough to see it and hoped I'd be able to share them with you at some point."

He flinched, as did she. "Me?"

He sighed and closed his eyes. "Yeah. I mean, Jack. Can I call you Jack, please? Just here?" She nodded. How could she refuse when it sounded so good coming from his lips?

"Only if I can go back to calling you Rhett."

"Hell yeah, I'll take it. Anyway, I've wanted to get to know you more since the day you woke up in my bed. I looked for you, like I said, but that didn't stop when I saw you in the hospital that first day."

"It…it didn't?" If she'd been struck mute before, that was nothing compared to how she felt now, with this knowledge.

"Of course not. It didn't even when I realized you'd be my rival for this job, nor when I found out you were carrying our child. If anything, I'm more drawn to you than ever before. And this isn't surprising to anyone as much as it is to me, believe me."

Everett leaned in, tucking himself behind her head. She rested against his chest, steadying a breath as the most calming feeling washed over her. After years of living side by side with fear and uncertainty, this was new and wholly unexpected. Heat built behind her eyes.

"So, what does this mean?" she asked. "I mean for work and you and me? Because I'm still going to fight for this job. You've seen where I live and why I need this."

He nodded. "I do. And I respect you for that more than you'll ever know, even if our situation is unconventional and complicated."

"That didn't answer my question," she said, laughing and nudging him with her shoulder. "We're having a baby and competing for a job. Calling us complicated is a little understated."

He exhaled deeply. She breathed in his scent, committing it to memory for a time she might be forced to live without it.

After a prolonged silence where she worried he'd forgotten her original question, he sat facing her.

"Okay. Hear me out and let me finish while I have the cojones to say this. Promise you'll listen to my whole idea before you jump in?" He was grinning like he knew exactly how hard that would be for her.

"Fine. But make it quick. I'm going to have to pee in a few minutes."

He nodded and dove in. "I want you to move in here." She opened her mouth, but he only had to shoot her a look for her to recall the stupid promise she'd made. She mimed sealing her lips, but wasn't sure how he thought this would be a good idea. "Anyway, I want you to move in here and get out of a place that is actively trying to make you leave anyway. Besides, what are you going to do in two months when you have an arm full of groceries and have to hike up four flights of stairs? Six months from now?"

He had a point, one she'd already considered. But moving in with the man who she was one part rival with and two parts attracted to? Was that a good idea?

You're already having a baby with him.

"It will let me take care of you, too. Both of you. Not in the 'you're an invalid' way, but I can drive you to doctor's appointments and make you healthy meals when you're too tired to cook. It's the least I can do, and besides, it gets me what I want, too."

"I think I know what that is," she finally admitted. At this point, she had to tell him; agreeing to live with him without disclosing that she was fighting for the job assuming he'd have an astronomical payout and could go back to practicing medicine for the F1 or rodeo teams was unfair at best.

"You do?" he asked. He took her hands in his. "I'm so glad. That makes this so much easier." The gentle way he gazed down at her made her wonder if they were talking about the same thing.

"Are you talking about the trust fund?" she

asked. The shadow that flitted across his face said no, he wasn't. *Oh no...*

"Did my brother tell you?" he growled, pulling away from her. The storm on his features was wild, untamed. It scared and captivated her at the same time. Why did he change so suddenly? What was the story there?

"No, he didn't. I just thought maybe it's our answer to the challenge between us. That if you take that, the job won't be something we're fighting over at least."

The hurricane of anguish calmed to a tropical storm. "I get it. And I hadn't considered that aspect of my inheritance. But, Jack, it's so complicated. I wish I could tell you I'll do that, that I can bow out of the job search and take this route, but that would mean giving in to a man I've worked hard to put out of my life, and I don't know if I can do that. But I'll try, for you."

Her heart swelled. He'd really do that for her? This man was intent on continuing to shock the hell out of her, wasn't he?

Rhett sighed and her heart lurched. This man had his own trauma to work through. Maybe they'd be good for one another, these two souls who had never learned what care and support should look like.

"No. I don't need that. We'll figure it out. But what happened? I know I'm not your person, but you can still talk to me, Rhett. I'm sorry if I ever made you feel like that wasn't true. I was wrapped up in my own fear." And she still was, but the worst was over; Rhett knew about the pregnancy and they were talking through the rest calmly. Her nervous system relaxed while her passion went into overdrive.

She tried to tame it to no avail, especially when he answered, "I'll tell you at some point—just not tonight. I want tonight to be about figuring us out."

"Okay. I can do that. I still think your idea is ridiculous. What was the one thing you wanted, by the way? I cut you off with the worst possible answer about what I thought you meant."

"Oh, yeah. All I want is time with you as you grow our tiny human, Jack. I want to get to know you and see how this…unconventional start to bringing a kid in the world is gonna work with you. I mean, isn't this usually why people date? To figure out their compatibility if they want to start a family together?"

A family. Two words that had eluded Jack her whole life. But somehow, she'd made one now, albeit unconventionally, as Rhett pointed out.

"I thought people dated to have good sex," she teased, deflecting from the sudden turn in seriousness.

"True. And to that end, since we aren't, you

know, actually dating, I have a spare room so you don't feel weird sharing a bed with me. Though if you ever feel like you'd like to bring sex into this again, my door is always open to you."

He winked and she was so thankful for the long flowing pants she wore that he couldn't see the flood of moisture that pooled in her panties when he mentioned bringing sex back to their "arrangement." There was something so magnetic about Rhett that she couldn't keep her good sense in her pants where it belonged. It wasn't just her physical attraction to him, either. No, this went deeper, to how he spoke to her and saw her.

That worried her more than just wanting to go to bed with the guy again. Which meant this idea was crazy, right?

"What about dating other people? You and I don't want a real relationship, right?"

There was a slight pause before Rhett answered. She tried not to read into it.

"No, we're still the same where that is concerned. But I don't need to date right now anyway. I've got a job, a baby and her mother to care for, and a brother to repair a relationship with. The last thing I need is another complication."

Jack tried not to be hurt at how he'd called her and their baby a "complication," but at least he'd joined her in calling the baby a *her*.

"What about what people at the hospital will think?"

"I don't really care about any of their opinions. This is bigger than everyone." Bigger than his brother's influence over his life? Jack found that hard to believe. "Bigger than Mack's opinion, too. He's got his own…challenges with Lainey."

It was as if Rhett had read her mind. It also seemed as if he was aware of his brother and Lainey's similar predicament, even if the circumstances were different. At least those two had a history of being together to rely on. Rhett and Jack barely knew one another.

This plan of his will help with that.

"I know about them, by the way," she said. If it turned out Rhett didn't, she could always pretend she meant that they were seeing one another in secret while they figured out what it all meant.

"About the…" Rhett's gaze shot to her abdomen and there was no guesswork needed. The brothers had to have talked. Did Mack know Rhett knew about his own pregnancy? Gosh, this was seven degrees of complicated, wasn't it?

"Yes. Lainey told me in confidence. She's also the one who slipped up with me about the trust."

Rhett smiled. "I've always liked Lainey. Partly because only she can get through that thick skull of my brother's. She's also a helluva doc, like you. I hope those two figure out a way not to screw it up this time. Anyone can see they're great together." Jack agreed, a hint of jealousy tugging at her heart. "But anyway, I'm glad you two have each other. It's kinda weird, isn't it? That two cousins will be born so close together?"

"It is. Thanks for talking through this with me, Rhett."

He took her hands again, this time kissing them. Then he gently guided her to a comfy kitchen chair and directed her to sit while he started cooking for her. How could she refuse?

"So does that mean you'll do it?"

"Sit?" she asked. He laughed.

"No, goofball. Move in here. It's got an elevator and killer view, not to mention an in-home chef." He flipped the eggs in his pan. "And you'll save on rent so you can put it toward a car for the baby, and I'll be around to help if you need it. Starting with talking to Mack so we can get you into the new birthing clinic. Lainey went and raved about it."

She was running out of reasons to say no to what seemed like a near-perfect scenario.

Yeah, near perfect if you are willing to settle for half a life. You're really willing to move in with a man who has openly admitted that love is off the table for him?

She was. After all, what did she know about love, aside from the fairy tale she'd been fed as a child? The reality was darker. To her, love only meant betrayal and a blanket under which to shove transgressions and guilt and other awful things. Maybe this was better. She'd get to live her own life without the trappings of a relationship, and get some perks of living with a beautiful man.

Why did her body have to go weak at the knees when she thought of one of those "perks"? This was going to be so dangerous, wasn't it?

At least, for the first time in her adulthood, there was room for more than just work in her life, after all… *Maybe.* Only if she kept her gaze facing forward and didn't do anything to jeopardize her job, which was, in the end, the only thing she could actually count on.

Because Rhett seemed like a good man, like an incredibly giving partner, especially when he had a million reasons not to be, but what about when times got tough and she really needed him? Would he be able to be the shoulder she needed to rest her weary head on?

Without knowing, she looked up at the man who'd captivated her body and heart and nodded.

"Yes," she said before she lost her nerve. "I'll move in with you." And then she sent up a prayer to the universe that she hadn't just damned herself by making a deal that seemed all too good to be true.

CHAPTER SEVEN

RHETT GOT UP and went for a jog around Lady Bird Lake. He didn't think he'd ever get sick of the reflection of the city off its water, the kind greetings from other runners and walkers, tourists and locals alike. Austin wasn't on his radar most of his life, but he was glad the pull of family and his last contract with the F1 circuit landed him there.

It felt like home.

Part of that was the place that he headed back to, his legs pumping faster the closer he got to his apartment. Sure, the location and overall place were fabulous—more than he had any right to ask for—but it wasn't the building or view that drew him back, made him feel like he had a home for the first time in his adult life.

It was Jack. She'd only had a few meager belongings, a result, she'd told him, of running from her first marriage when her husband's abuse had grown deadly. What she did bring with her, and what he took her shopping to replace, made his place into a sanctuary. Now, he rushed through his days, eager to get back to her, and this run was no exception.

His lungs burned under the strain. Finally, he rounded the corner and saw a familiar shape in the kitchen window. His pulse skyrocketed, and not because of the exertion of the exercise.

Jack. God, she was beautiful, and was she… was she singing and dancing? He slowed to a stop and watched her for a moment. She was unabashed and confidently belting something he couldn't hear, but damn was it a pleasure to watch. She wore a baggy T-shirt, but he knew from experience that was all she had on.

How anyone had hurt that woman—how anyone hurt any person they claimed to love—was out of his scope of understanding, but it started a fire in his belly just thinking about it. That woman up there was precious and had been even before he knew she was carrying his child.

His phone went off and he begrudgingly pulled himself from watching Jack to see who it was. His frown was immediate.

"Hey, Mack, what's up?" His older brother hadn't exactly taken the news that Rhett and Jack were moving in together well. In his opinion, it was a guaranteed way to make sure the two of them not only imploded at work, but drove one another away at home, too. Per Mack's sage wisdom, raising a kid together when you were playing house with someone you had no intention of marrying was creating a "false environment" that could only erode under the weight of the truth over time.

God, Mack could be so sanctimonious sometimes.

In truth, living with Jack had been a breeze so far, even if it had only been a few days. They had almost matching schedules since Mack and the HR team were observing them during surgeries and shifts with other patients, so they traveled in and back together. He cooked and when she wasn't sick, Jack insisted on cleaning up. They laughed, played music while they cooked, and at the end of the night, they read their books on his oversize sofa until Jack inevitably fell asleep on her side.

His secret favorite was when her feet would migrate over and tuck under his legs while she dozed. He craved to be closer to her, to ask her to curl up in his lap so he could rub her head and help her sleep, but that wasn't his decision.

He'd promised to keep his distance unless and until Jack wanted more. There'd been moments he'd thought she might. When he walked by her and let her know he was there with a hand on the small of her back, she leaned into his touch. But she'd gone to bed every night alone. He was dying, wondering if maybe his brother was right.

Was it a disaster to expect to raise a baby with a woman he cared for but couldn't commit to?

What did she think? On one hand, she seemed content with their arrangement, but did that mean she also didn't want a relationship? That she was fine without any promises of commitment or… love?

Why does it matter? You laid out your terms and we both agreed to them.

His inner critic sounded an awful lot like Mack.

But it wasn't wrong. Why did it matter so much what Jack wanted out of him? He was maxed out on what he could do, what he could offer.

Because you care about her, and like it or not, Mack's right. You're playing house with her. If it looks like a relationship, sounds like one and feels like one…

He didn't let himself finish that thought. Not here, not now. Not with her close enough to touch and tempt him more than he already was. The thing about it, about the question that had been sitting on his tongue for days now—*What are we?*—was that he'd never asked it before. And he wanted to know.

Ugh. At least he had some time to think about it when he went in today. They weren't scheduled together that evening, since she was pulling a double shift the next day, one in each of the new sites. His time for that was the day after, meaning three days they wouldn't see one another. He already wanted that time to pass, for them to get back to their new normal.

What did that mean?

"Rhett, you there?"

"Yeah. Sorry, just got back from a run and I'm stretching," he said. It was sort of true. He was stretching his calves along the apartment's curb. And he considered his thinking through what was going on with his feelings for Jack a stretch of his normal MO.

"Well, I need your full attention. Are you and Jack together?"

Rhett pinched the bridge of his nose. "No. I'm still outside."

"She isn't answering her phone so I called you." Rhett made his way to the door and walked in. Sure enough, music was playing loud enough to drown out any ringtone.

"Yeah, she probably had the phone on silent," Rhett said, smiling as he watched Jack using it as a microphone while she danced to some new song from the radio. When she whirled and caught him staring, she turned a bright shade of crimson, her cheeks looking like his shoulders after a run in the summer sun.

"Fine. Can you bring her in when you come in later? One of the peds cases from the new site was moved here for bed space there, and I could use Jack's expertise."

"Do you need us now?" Rhett asked. He made his way to Jack and wrapped her in a hug. She buried her face in his chest, not seeming to care that he was sweaty. A hint at the answer he'd been searching for tickled the back of his throat.

"I'm mortified," she whispered.

"Shh," he said. He kissed her on the forehead and squeezed her tight against him, inhaling her scent. How did she still smell so delectable in the morning? "You're beautiful."

She stepped back and he blanched. Shit. Had he just kissed her? Then told her she was beautiful? His feelings had been sitting in the periphery, but he'd pushed them down where they couldn't get in the way. So what, they'd leaked out?

That's what he got for wondering about the nature of their blossoming...relationship. *Friendship.*

Even as he thought that last word, he was aware how shallow it sounded compared to how he felt.

Shit.

"Sorry," he whispered back. "I—"

"Rhett? Good grief. I feel like I'm talking to a wall." Mack was still on the line.

"Sorry, Mack," Rhett said, turning away from Jack. "Anyway, do you need us now?"

The exasperated sigh on the other line was so

typically Mack. “Like I already said, no. Come in when you’re scheduled and thank her for me.”

“Of course.”

Rhett couldn’t get off the phone fast enough. He wheeled around, expecting to find Jack packing her bags and heading back to her apartment. Not that he’d blame her. They’d flirted the line between friends and…more, but never acted on it.

So when he found himself face-to-face with her, her bottom lip tucked between her teeth and wide eyes gazing up at him, he was stunned silent.

“What did Mack want?”

Everett had to clear his throat twice to find the words he searched for.

“He wants me to bring you in with me. They have a consult for you from the trauma site. I guess he tried calling you but you didn’t answer.” She didn’t even glance down at her phone. Instead, she took a step toward him.

“Do we need to leave now?” He shook his head, afraid to breathe in her scent and be rendered dumb. “Good.”

Then, she wrapped her arms around him again and pressed her head against his chest as she had before. When he didn’t react—how could he without worrying he’d break whatever spell had her touching him, hugging him—she nuzzled his chin with the top of her head.

He thought he understood, but he pleaded silently, *please don't let me be wrong.*

He kissed the top of her head and felt her nod against him. Everett pulled back, as did Jack. He searched her eyes, finding only promise. He bent down and kissed her forehead again, all the while, pulling himself tighter against her.

Jack squeezed back and then tipped up on her toes to kiss him, this time on the lips. Fire like he'd only read about, heard rumors of, consumed him limb by limb. He opened his mouth and used his tongue to explore her mouth, teasing and tasting her in kind. When Jack moaned into his mouth, he exploded.

Where they'd started their kiss tentative and sweet, it grew in intensity, both of them pulling and pushing and arching into the other as if they'd both held back for far too long and couldn't any longer.

Everett's hands slid up Jack's baggy t-shirt, and he released a growl of lust when he discovered she wore neither a bra nor full panties. Instead, he traced the small of her back down until his hands met with a nanoscopic swathe of lace just above the top of her curvy backside.

"God damn, woman. You have no idea what you do to me." He cupped her butt and squeezed and she squealed with delight. If he didn't have the modicum of self-control he was clinging to, he'd have come right there.

She kissed his chest, tracing his pec muscle with her tongue, then moving across to the other and giving it the same treatment.

"Jack," he groaned. His voice was thick and almost unrecognizable. She sucked along his abdominal wall, nipping at him softly every so often. And then she was on her knees in front of him, sliding his running shorts over his hips and taking him in her mouth with one move he could barely follow, his brain was so scrambled. "You're killing me," he murmured as her lips teased his tip.

And that was all he could say as words were ripped from his chest and replaced by guttural groans and moans of pleasure such as he'd never known. Jack's right hand cupped his balls while the other one worked with her mouth over him, faster, tighter, until a pull in his lower stomach told him he was close to exploding.

His hands fisted in her hair and he didn't have to pull her closer; she found his base on her own and swallowed him whole with each dip of her head.

"Jack," he growled. She didn't stop, but instead tightened her grip and teased his tip with her tongue. "Ah, fuck. I'm gonna come," he said. She gave a small nod but didn't stop until he shot into her with everything he had. He shuddered as every last bit of him filled her, and she swallowed what he gave her.

His knees buckled and he collapsed on the floor beside her.

"Oh, I hope you're not done that easily," she said, straddling him. He was ready to reply that he needed a minute, maybe an hour to recuperate, when his erection sprang up like it hadn't just been sucked to completion. "That's a good boy," Jack said, stroking him.

"Dammit, Jack. You're either the devil in disguise or a witch. I can't be sure which."

She sat atop his length, teasing his tip with her center while she peppered his chest with kisses. She'd done the same thing the night they met, and he'd had the distinct feeling that she was calm personified. It wasn't as if other lovers hadn't kissed his chest, or hugged him tight, but there was something so delicate and intimate with how Jack touched him.

It was like each touch of her skin to his was intentional and embedded with emotion far beyond simple lust. No wonder the condom hadn't worked. It didn't stand a chance when all of him reacted to her in the way it did.

"I know we talked about this the night we met, but I haven't been with anyone but you in three years," she told him. "And I'm clear."

He nodded. "Me, too. You're my last partner, too." At that moment, he couldn't imagine taking on another partner ever again, but he kept that part to himself until he could make sense of what that meant to his self-imposed "no dating" rule.

The idea that she might choose another partner one day—likely would if they weren't a real couple—almost killed his erection, but he ignored the future and focused on the gorgeous half-naked woman on top of him. It was all he could ask for and more, and he planned on cherishing every last second.

She slid over him, and just like before, he filled her completely.

"Then since the form of birth control we used didn't work last time, we don't need to bother with a condom, do we?" She rocked back and forth and even though he'd just come, he felt the pull again.

Yeah, the devil or a witch. He didn't care either way as long as she kept doing what she was doing.

"No. No condom," he managed to say. It was a hoarse whisper that got swallowed by a gasp.

"God, you feel good, Jack." She rode him slow at first, much like their kiss, then bent over him, kissing him deeply, her tongue tangling with his.

Her breasts brushed against his chest, and he marveled at how full they were compared to when they'd first slept together. When she rocked over him, he took one of them in his mouth and sucked. Jack arched her back and cried out.

"Are you okay?" he asked. She gazed down at him with a smile on her face that was unlike any he'd seen on her yet. It was joy, pure and simple.

"I'm so good. Please don't stop. They're just more sensitive now." He obliged, cupping one breast while he sucked on the other. She picked up intensity as she moved over him. Each time she took him deeper, he could feel her tighten around him.

"I'm close," she cried out. "Everett—" Her arms trembled and he flipped her on her back without leaving her. "Yes, yes, please. Take me."

He could never take another direction in his life as long as she guided him with how to please her. Everett drove into her, reaching her core with each thrust. She cried out each time and gripped his hips tighter, driving his pace and depth. She felt so good, so goddamn perfect.

"I'm going to come with you," he said, the orgasm building. At this rate, it would be powerful enough to make the last one—which was earth-shattering enough—feel like nothing more than a flutter of butterflies.

"Please," she whispered. Her nails scraped down his back and she lifted her hips, taking more of him in somehow. He was sheathed, tip to base. "Please come with me. I'm… I'm there."

So was he. He felt the release in every limb, every cell of his body. Their bodies trembled as he turned her on her side and held her against him.

She exhaled and melted into the S-curve he'd made with his leg and torso, all the while kissing his chest. The kisses undid him and he pressed her tighter, unwilling to let her go. He refused to examine that too deeply. When her trembles turned to deep, soft breaths, he assumed she'd fallen asleep. That was, until she traced his chest muscles with the tip of her finger, sending warmth outward from each spot she touched.

"Well, that was…something," she said through giggles. It triggered a wave of his own laughter and before he knew it, they were both wiping tears from their cheeks. After what seemed like hours, but was probably mere minutes, they calmed and recovered their breath.

"It was definitely something," he said, and fought back another round of giggles. "I hope something good?"

The serious question seemed to sober her as well. She gazed up at him and nodded.

"Yes. Very. Complicated, maybe, but…good."

"That's an understatement on all accounts," he said, kissing her. "But I wouldn't mind doing it again from time to time."

She ran her fingers along his arm and back. "Mmm. Me, too. Like, in the next few minutes, if you're up for it." Jack nipped his bottom lip with her teeth and he laughed.

"Yeah, I think I could swing that." He deepened their kiss and as he did, he had a singular thought, aside from the insight that what they'd just shared was the best sexual experience of his life so far.

This. This is what can happen when you care for someone you sleep with. Complicated was a good word to describe it, but so was *peace. Home.*

Love?

Oh, no. As soon as his mind came up with the word, he wondered if it was true. He'd been forever changed by the woman in his arms and like it or not, there was nothing to do about it now. But was it that serious, that his body, in the throes of passion could come up with "love" as the answer to "what am I feeling?"

So, what does this mean if it is *love?* He wished he had an answer for that, specifically. Dating was hard for him, near impossible, even. But so was the opposite, where he'd be forced to walk away from Jack if he couldn't give her what she deserved.

And really, there wasn't a middle ground, was there? There was only one option as far as he could see. And it terrified him to his core.

Was "love" enough of a reason to make a go of something when his whole life he'd been running from that exact scenario? Was loving her possible if his singular goal was to build a world of his own, free from his family and other obligations that might complicate that?

What would it hurt to try?

That wasn't the worst idea. It's not as if by saying he wanted to date her that he was marrying her or anything. After all, they were having a baby together, sleeping together now, and they worked well as colleagues. How much of a stretch was it to build this life together? If it didn't work out, he could leave. Couples broke up all the time and still found a way to parent peacefully.

It wasn't exactly a plan, but it was a start. He liked Jack, whether or not he *loved* her. Either way, saying goodbye was untenable right now. He'd keep the rest of it close to his chest for now, but that didn't mean he couldn't start to show her how he felt and see how it went.

He kissed her, savoring the brine on her lips, a mix of them both that somehow tasted better than the wine they'd had the night they met. Before he knew it, their bodies were joined again, and he was as sated as a man had any right to be.

He knew the world was waiting to bite at their heels, stealing any and all of their newfound happiness. His brother, their jobs, the competition for the trauma doc position, his father…it all growled and barked outside his door.

He'd be damned if he was going to let that ruin

the moment, though. When his phone rang, he ignored it. Whatever was needed—work, patients, or his brother—could wait. Right now, he had all he needed in his arms, and he didn't want another darn thing.

Later, he'd wish he held on to this feeling, that he hadn't checked his email. Maybe then, things wouldn't have unraveled as quickly as they did.

CHAPTER EIGHT

JACK DIDN'T KNOW what hit her. It was as if a rogue wave of oxytocin had slammed into her, and she'd fallen into its depths. Everything under the surface was hazy and dreamlike, and she wasn't sure she wanted to come back to reality.

She'd found out she was pregnant and thought it was the end of everything she wanted in life. Her independence, her career and her chance at love with a partner who wanted what she did.

Instead, everything was the opposite. Being independent was easy if you didn't have to grow a human and go to work and cook yourself healthy meals. Living with Rhett was a dream come true. Right now, he cooked, which she loved since she was usually too tired to come up with anything creative and healthy that would support the growing life inside her.

She'd tried to help with dishes each night, but he'd shooed her away, citing too many cooks in the kitchen. So, she'd chatted with him to help pass the time, filling him in on everything in her life before the cataclysmic event he was already aware of.

Every now and then, he'd come over and kiss her, or splash water on her, eliciting giggles she hadn't let loose in—well, she couldn't recall how long.

When it came to her career, she was happy, too. She'd shared a couple cases with Rhett since they'd expanded their…extracurriculars to include casual sex. Not only hadn't their affair negatively affected her concentration, it almost seemed to have increased her focus.

She worked alongside Rhett like they'd been colleagues for years, not weeks. Even Mack noticed, complimenting them both the previous afternoon when they were grabbing a bite to eat. Thankfully, Rhett had just snuck a kiss behind a partition and they were walking half a body's length apart so nothing looked suspicious.

"You two do good work together," Mack said. Rhett had rolled his eyes, but Jack took the words for what they were—a sweet gesture, an olive branch even, from a man who had a complicated relationship with his family, much as Rhett did. Though she had to admit that the more time Mack spent with Lainey, the kinder and more outgoing he became, even to Rhett.

"Any chance you'll hire us both then?" Rhett

asked. To be fair, Jack had thought it, but she'd never have had the courage to say it aloud.

"We'll see what funding will allow. A private donor is funding the off-site clinics, and there may be an opportunity there. It's dicey, though, and I won't have an answer for a few weeks, I'm afraid."

She understood. When he was out of sight, Rhett snuck another kiss, this time on the lips.

"Rhett," she'd said, chastising him. It was adorable, and darn if her stomach didn't flip a thousand ways from Sunday. But it was so inappropriate. She wasn't sure she was comfortable with public displays of affection, but not for the reasons he thought.

She didn't want the scrutiny of being seen romantically with the boss's brother, and sure, she also didn't want anything to pull focus from the good work she was doing. But mostly, they hadn't spoken about what this did to their unconventional relationship, both agreeing to just "see where it went."

Until they could chat, she didn't want to provide answers to folks' queries. That was to say, she didn't mind a secret kiss or two away from prying eyes, but she'd rather not invite questions she couldn't answer.

And then there was the idea of being in love with a partner who wanted what she did. She wasn't so naive as to say that she and Rhett had turned a corner there. In fact, the one negative aspect of their relationship was that they hadn't spoken about their change in status since she'd kissed him, igniting this whirlwind passion between them.

But the possibility was there, at least. She could feel it. How could it not be when they worked so well together, when they supported one another so completely?

Take that afternoon for example. He was taking the back part of the day off to go with her to the new clinic so they could meet with an ob-gyn about establishing care. He'd made the appointment and taken the time off so he could find out how to care for her during the pregnancy, all without her even making the suggestion.

A knock on the hospital locker room door roused her from her daydreaming, bringing her back to the surface where reality awaited her. Luckily, reality just then was a meeting with another colleague to see how her and Rhett's baby was doing.

She opened the door to find Rhett there with a flower made from blue paper towels they used in surgical rooms.

"What's this?" she asked, taking it and pretending to sniff.

"It's a clean one," he said, winking at her.

"Gosh, I hope so, but…why?"

It was such a sweet gesture, but like everything Rhett did, she found herself asking *why*?

"I'm excited to see the doctor and hopefully our little bean. Thought I'd share my appreciation for you in letting me come along. That's all."

That was all? That was *everything.*

"Of course. You're her dad. You're always invited." A nagging intrusive thought crept in. Would she actually always want him there? If they stopped…doing whatever it was they were doing and went back to colleagues and roommates, would this be healthy for her to treat him like a partner?

She didn't know, nor was she ready to act on future worries. The therapist she'd seen after leaving Orin had cautioned against that, and for the most part, she'd been right so far that it was a dangerous and lonely way to live.

That said, lonely was better than one alternative. At least Rhett didn't seem remotely capable of turning into a monster like Orin.

"Anyway, should we get going? It sounds like they're keeping busy. Reynolds texted and said they have a full waiting room of walk-ins."

"For OB care?" Jack asked. Rhett nodded and walked alongside her, his hand brushing against hers. It sent shivers down her spine.

"Yep. Same at the new peds and trauma site, too."

"I wish I could help out there. I think I could do a lot of good," Jack admitted. She hadn't expressed that particular wish out loud, but it felt right sharing it with Rhett. What could come of it, she wasn't sure, but maybe she should take a page from his book and just ask Mack.

They made it outside, and Rhett tucked them inside a waiting car. Once they were in the back of the rideshare vehicle, he kissed her long and deep.

"I think you could, too," he said, pulling back and resting his forehead against hers. "I wish Mack would get his head out of his…well, you know, and think of hiring from within the hospital. If he did, he'd realize you're a perfect fit. You've got the experience and the background to make a difference with these families who use the clinic."

"Thanks, Rhett." That was the most seen she'd felt by another human in her life. She kissed him softly on the lips, marveling at how much peace it brought her. He was like coming home to a warm bed and meal after days out in a storm. "Do you really think Mack would hire us both like you teased him about the other day?" she asked.

Rhett shrugged and pulled her tight into him.

"I don't know. My brother is reasonable, but also pragmatic as hell. He'll do it if he can see the black numbers at the bottom of a balance sheet, but if you bring emotion into the equation, no, I don't think we can count on him doing what's right just because he likes us both. Unfortunately," he added. She wiggled away, but he held her tighter. "No come here."

He wrapped both arms around her, cradling her stomach. As a pregnant lady, she should wear a seat belt, but the rideshare van seemed to have a broken one where she was sitting. Rhett's arm around her made her feel safe, like he'd protect her if anything happened. Luckily the clinic was a short ride away and they made it no problem.

"I'll be in the area grabbing lunch if you get done in the next hour and need a lift back," the driver said.

Rhett took the business card he proffered and tipped him before escorting her into the new Austin Memorial Family Birth Center.

"This is so nice," Jack commented as they walked inside. The walls were a pale cerulean, with a mural on one of a quote in elegant script. It read, "All families are welcome here," and was surrounded by animals and kids of every race and ethnicity and size and shape. It was perfect.

"Yeah, the design team did a fabulous job. Austin Memorial is the most inclusive system in the southwest by a landslide. It's one of the things I know Mack is proud of. One of the things our mom left us."

"I'd have liked to meet her."

Rhett smiled down at her, his hand discreetly on her lower back while they waited to check in. "She'd have loved to meet you. You two would have been thick as thieves, actually. I don't think I'd have trusted either of you to go into a bookstore together, though. You'd have both walked out with more books than you could carry."

Jack laughed. "Oh, if that was her guilty pleasure, then yes, we would have had a good time together."

While they waited to be called back to an exam room, they talked about books Jack loved, about what books Everett used to read before his day job became too stressful to keep up with a whole novel without losing who the characters were and where the plot was headed. It was odd being on the patient end of things, but it wasn't stressful as she'd worried, being in an OB office, largely because it was near impossible to be stressed around Rhett.

Sure, in the beginning that wasn't true. But it wasn't Rhett so much as the circumstances that were in the way. Now, something had shifted. They'd come to some sort of unspoken agreement and even the fact that they were still rivals for the same job didn't worry her. She would be okay, she knew that now.

Rhett was a big part of that. He held her hand, even though technically, these people were their colleagues. No one knew them, though, not really. They were both too new to Austin Memorial. His hand in hers felt like peace, and his passionate curiosity about her was so damn sexy. The combination was pure relaxation and a limited concern about what their appointment would yield.

The only nagging worry was whether he felt the same way she did. There were times she felt as if he saw her clear as day and moved not only with, but toward her. Today was one of those days.

There were other moments, though, where a war waged in his features, as if he were battling demons she couldn't see. He'd clam up and though yes, he always came back to her, those moments worried her.

"Jacqueline Elliot?" a nurse asked. Jacqueline waved and stood. "Welcome to AMFBC. How are you feeling?"

"Great," Jack said, following the nurse. Rhett was right behind her, a steady presence keeping her nerves at bay. "I feel pregnant, believe it or not."

Already, she could tell her own energy was waning, her stomach showing off a slight distention where it used to be flat. To anyone else, it would appear she'd had a big lunch, but she could feel the difference in her body. Even though, compared to the women in the waiting room who looked about ready to go into labor, she was barely showing.

"That makes sense. It says here you're already almost nine weeks pregnant, so you're probably experiencing some bloating and tiredness, right?"

Jack nodded. The tiredness was an understatement. She found it hard to keep her eyes open past seven anymore. Only one thing helped to keep her awake, and even that wasn't a guarantee.

"She also eats in smaller amounts and urinates with greater frequency," Rhett added.

Jack had been sunburned once in her life, a gift, considering how much she basked in the outdoors with a book any time she got a chance. But that sunburn had felt like her cheeks were on fire for three straight days.

And that was exactly how she felt now, with Rhett talking about her bathroom habits.

"Can we please not talk about my urination?" she hissed, hiding her face with shame.

He laughed and kissed her head. "Sweetie, I'm not gonna go announcing to everyone at the bar that you pee a lot, but I think the doc will need to know."

She didn't disagree, but hearing the man she was sleeping with, working alongside and having a baby with talking about her pee still wasn't comfortable.

"Fine," she mumbled. "Yes, I pee more."

Inside the exam room, everything became very real. The OB introduced herself and spoke very highly of Mack's plans for the center. She assured Rhett and Jack that their showing up to the exam together was top secret, and they knew she meant it. HIPAA laws prevented physicians from sharing information about patients with people who weren't approved by the patient.

"Do you want to see the baby?" she asked once the preliminary questions were out of the way.

"Yes, please," Rhett and Jack said at the same time. They shared a laugh as well, and when her hands began to shake, he took them in his.

"We've got this," he said. Gazing up at him, she knew they did. Whatever came their way, they would tackle together.

Wow, she thought. *How much has changed in such a short time.*

The doctor prepped Jack for the procedure, then moments later displayed the ultrasound image on the monitor, and both Rhett and Jack gasped. A tear slid down her cheek as she watched the black and white image come to life before them. Though the body could barely be considered as much, with its bulbous center and four little sprouts that would become arms and legs one day soon, it was beautiful.

My angel. It was hers, something no one could take away.

Rhett squeezed her hand and even though she was filled with intense longing for the man who had given her this, she also realized he was the one exception to her thought. He could take the child from her if they split up.

A shiver of dread coursed through her.

Don't borrow worry. She repeated the mantra, but hadn't life shown her that even when things seemed to be going well, it could all be taken from her? Exercising control when and where she could was paramount to keeping herself and her baby safe.

"Are you okay?" Rhett asked. There he went, recognizing her infinitesimal shifts in mood and addressing them. Hopefully, her fears would never come to fruition. What she wanted most was to build a life and family with this man, but that meant they needed to finally talk about their living and intimate situation.

"I'm okay. This is just a lot, that's all. But it's beautiful."

He squeezed her shoulder and bent down to kiss her. "It is. What do you need from me?" he asked.

She was touched at his question. The OB cleaned up Jack's stomach.

"Everything looks great. I'll see you both in a month." She left, giving them privacy for her to get dressed.

"I think we need to talk about what this all means," she started.

He nodded, smiling. "Of course. But I'm not worried. We're going to be fine." Oh, why couldn't she share his optimism?

Because you're coming off a horrific relationship you had to leave to save your own life. Give yourself grace.

It was her therapist's words, but her own voice she heard. She could do that, could give herself grace. But something told her she was running out of time, that they were headed for a cliff and she couldn't save herself and her baby if they didn't slow down or shift their heading. Or at least know that he'd be there to catch her if they careened off together.

We can only control ourselves, not other people. More therapist-speak, but not untrue either. She could trust what Rhett told and showed her, but in the end, it was up to her.

"And," she added, "I want to make some sort of agreement, on paper I mean."

"What kind of agreement?"

She swallowed, her throat dry. "Custody. I want to know that if we stop doing whatever this is, we won't try to take our child away from the other person."

The look of horror on Rhett's open mouth, his smile flipped on its head and his brows arched in pain, told her she'd crossed a line. But it wasn't about her, it was to protect her child. It had to be said.

"I would never do that to you, Jack. I know you've been through hell and if I could take that pain away, I'd do whatever it took. All I can do moving forward is protect you and make sure no one else hurts you. But I can guarantee it won't be me."

She bristled. Orin, in his vows, had sworn to protect her every day he was alive, and in the end, he'd caused more harm than anyone else in her life. How was she ever supposed to trust those words again, even all dressed up in a package as delectable as Rhett.

"You can't make those kinds of guarantees, but we can make them regarding our child. That's how you can help me. If I think she can be taken from me—" She choked on a sob.

"Shh," he said, rubbing her back. "I'll sign whatever agreement you want, as long as you will allow me to be in her life as well."

"Of course. I'd never keep her from you." She relaxed, knowing he wouldn't fight her on this. Rhett was a good man, and would be an amazing father. On that, she could put her trust.

They held each other tightly as he called the number on the card for the driver. In minutes he was there, and though it'd only been an hour since they'd gotten a ride to the center, everything had changed.

Rhett and Jack held hands, his arm still wrapped around her while they made their way back to the hospital where she had to start an evening shift. He'd taken the side of the vehicle without the seat belt this time, arguing that she needed to keep herself and the baby safe. It was sweet how much he cared, especially after being so adamant about not wanting kids.

She wasn't excited about leaving Rhett's side, not when there was so much on the cusp of being discovered and realized between them. But the bottom line remained. He wasn't taking the inheritance, and she wasn't giving up on the job. As of now, she hadn't asked about the clinic position. Therefore, she still had to show up and keep building the life for her and her child, as if she only had herself to count on.

"We're going to be parents," he whispered, kissing her ear. She beamed, the heat from earlier creeping back. This time, she didn't mind as much. Especially when it led to desire flooding right behind it.

"We are. We should probably talk more about that, too. Like if she'll go to preschool and if we're breastfeeding… And…" She trailed off as his kisses migrated to her neck, then behind her ear, as his hands fisted in her hair.

"And?" he asked, his breath warm where his lips had dampened her skin.

"And we should talk about this...this thing we're doing."

Rhett's hands slipped along the inside of her thigh. It was tempting to give into the physical passion this man brought out in her, a temptation she'd given in to a dozen times the past few days. But the voice in her head wouldn't be silenced.

They needed to slow things down, do them right so they were there for their child—and each other, hopefully—when the time came.

"Oh, you mean this thing?" he asked. His voice was husky, a perk of his want for her since the deep rasp turned her on even more. God, he knew just how to turn her heavy thoughts into effervescent bubbles of desire.

"Yes," she whispered. This man was going to be the death of her.

"Maybe later. I'm busy right now." His finger traced her panty line, then brushed against her sex. She was wet in seconds.

She giggled. "But you can't do this. We're in a public vehicle." She glanced up at the rearview mirror, but the driver didn't seem to be watching them. In fact, the terrified look on his face—

"Watch out!" he cried at the same time their car was hit almost head-on.

The seat belt locked in place, and Jack screamed

with pain as it felt like it was ripping her in half. Her head slammed against the window and the last thing she saw was the father of her baby, a man she cared for more than anyone in the world, as he flew into the front of the car since he wasn't wearing a seat belt.

With the sound of a crunch as his body slammed into glass and metal, she blacked out.

CHAPTER NINE

EVERETT ROLLED OVER, and all the bliss, the calm, the unbridled joy he'd accumulated by kissing Jack—finally—evaporated when he checked the time on his phone. He still had a few hours until his medical exam that would clear him to go back to work, but the ten texts and two voicemails made him wonder if he'd missed something.

He wasn't on call, and neither was Jack. They'd taken Rhett and Jack off surgeries while they both healed, but a few days into feeling better, he'd been stir-crazy and craving the call that they'd been medically cleared. At least the exam today should finalize things. Until then, he'd just keep kissing Jack, being thankful that their baby was okay.

When they'd crashed—

Rhett shuddered. He still felt the injury in his right shoulder, but he'd been lucky the guys in the F1 circuit taught him how to brace for impact if there was a crash. The thing that kept him up at night, and had for almost a full week, was the sickening sound of the scream Jack gave as she was trapped by the force of the seat belt across her abdomen.

He'd come out of the wreckage sore and needing a CT for head injuries that might have occurred, but Jack, even seatbelted in, had incurred the worst of the wreck. For starters, the car that had slammed into them had been going double the speed limit, and when it lost control and veered into oncoming traffic, it'd been Jack's side of the car that was hit.

Even when he could fall asleep, Rhett was haunted by the revolving images of Jack unconscious on a gurney, being hooked up to tubes and wires like she was just another patient while he watched on from afar, trying to pretend his whole world wasn't in that bed, and lastly, the faint whisper of a heartbeat that faded into nothingness when the OB had come in to check on their baby.

It had come back, thank goodness, but for a solid half a minute, Rhett had recalled the utter bliss he'd felt at the beginning of the day when he'd met their little one for the first time juxtaposed against the fear of losing her and her mother in the same heartbreaking instant. The canyon between those two emotions was almost insurmountable.

"Where'd you go?" Jack asked. Her voice was

still hoarse from the intubation, but she sounded—and looked—better every day.

"Sorry, just—"

"Thinking about it again?" she asked. He nodded, except if he told her the truth, that he rarely thought of anything else, she'd worry about him, and he couldn't have that on top of everything else.

One more reality had occurred to him the night before last, as if the horror show of losing his—what, girlfriend? Mother of his child?—wasn't enough.

Defining what Jack was to him was another problem for another time. The problem with thinking he was losing Jack was what those sounds and smells brought back, namely the moment he'd almost walked away from the F1 circuit forever. Being in this job in any capacity brought the carnage to his feet at work, but loving and caring for people meant anything they endured trauma-wise was laid at his front door to sift through.

"Hey," Jack said, kissing his chest. "I'm here and I'm fine. We're fine," she added, placing both their hands on her stomach. He fought the urge to press her against him and never let go. Each day, that feeling only got worse.

Today was by far the most intense as they were both heading out of the apartment for the first time since being released from Austin Memorial.

She'd been on temporary bed rest for a few days, then resting at home a few more, but she'd insisted on going in to get cleared for work. Mack and Rhett had both vocalized their objections—the first major thing they'd agreed on—so she'd gone around them both and gotten a third opinion. He'd keep an eye on her, and wasn't above pulling rank as the father of their child if she seemed tired or overworked.

On a positive note, a mysterious donor had funded further changes to the new sites, freeing up the budget a bit. According to Mack, that didn't quite equate to a second full-time position opening up, but it did mean he could extend the "observation period" a little so they could heal and spend some time helping to get the other sites fully up and running so patients had less wait time before being seen by a provider.

However, if a full-time, permanent position became available at one of the sites, he knew without a shadow of a doubt Jack would want it. No doubt that was the reason she was so desperate to get back to work and prove herself.

Not that he blamed her; he'd likely do the same thing. Hell, wasn't he, really? If he caved and gave in to his father's demands for the inheritance, Jack was right—he could seek out work anywhere. But he wanted life on his terms, so how could he fault Jack for wanting the same?

Will those "terms" include each other?

He still didn't know that answer. Each time his heart asked, his mind answered in opposition. Vice versa if it was his brain asking the question. He just couldn't get the two to align.

"I know, but that was too close for comfort. I hope you know how much I care about you, Jack. That if anything happened to you, I'd—"

He'd what? The thing was, he couldn't ever finish that sentence. Nor could he articulate how he felt about her, not in the larger sense, anyway. He knew he cared about her, but beyond that, he was still the same person with the same messed up past.

Riding the line between keeping her from it and holding her tight and protecting her from the rest of the world seemed to be impossible.

His phone buzzed again.

"Where are you?" Mack asked.

Home! Resting from the accident, he wanted to shout, but his brother knew that. So, what was Mack getting at? Surely his brother would have said something about him coming back earlier when they'd spoken? He flipped through the rest of his texts, which were all from Mack, of course. They varied in severity, from a benign Call me back when you get this, to a more serious Listen, are you okay? Call me back, Rhett. I want to get you both cleared so we can get Jack's opinion on something.

Well, that was a shift from Mack's earlier position about keeping Jack home another couple days.

Finally, they ended with the calls, which were verbal lashings for Everett not picking up.

The last message was over two minutes long, but it began with, "Where the hell are you? At this point I just want to know you two are safe. Please call me back."

"Come on," he muttered.

"Mmm. What's that?" Jack asked, rolling over and kissing him.

"Nothing. Just my brother being an overprotective ass." He said it with some sarcasm, but really, he had to admit it was nice to have Mack in his corner again. They were starting to feel like...like *family*.

Jack laughed, then winced. He knew her ribs were still causing her pain when she breathed deep or laughed. That seat belt had saved her life, but it'd also almost killed their infant with the pressure from the strap around her abdomen.

"That sounds familiar," she said, getting up from the bed. His gaze stayed pinned to her while she maneuvered around the mattress and headed into the bathroom. Technically, her bed rest had ended days ago, but he still got so nervous about her moving around. They'd had as close a call as they could have and still walk away from it. "You're not exactly willing to relinquish control, either."

"What do you mean?" he asked, following her into the bathroom. They'd moved into the same room before the accident, and never shifted back. Thank goodness, too. He didn't think he could be parted from her and not worry the night away. What the actual hell was he supposed to do when she went back to work full time?

"I mean, you're in the bathroom when I am, you're in bed when I come to bed, you follow me to the shower when you've already rinsed off. You're like a golden retriever."

"I'll take that as a compliment."

She raised her brows at him, but smiled, still. "Okay, dear. Whatever you need." She looked at her watch before taking it off to shower and gasped. "God, we really wasted half a day, didn't we? We were going to do laundry before the meeting, but it's nearly noon."

"I wouldn't call the day wasted." They'd kissed and he'd even trailed the length of her body with his lips, searching for places to bring her pleasure enough that she could forget the pain for even a little while. He'd paused to look at the long blue-black bruise across her abdomen for the briefest of seconds before her hands fisted in his hair and pushed him lower till he reached her core.

He'd kissed her there until she cried out with pleasure. The sound was brought on by pure joy, but it was still so similar to the one she'd released during the crash that it made him nauseated just as she came with a final cry.

They'd fallen asleep at some point, which was good because his body had needed a break from the exertion; they'd made love one whole night through just before the accident, but so much had happened since, that he could barely keep his eyes open for more than four hours at a stretch.

He might have to talk to Mack about limited hours if he was cleared for work—for both of them. He didn't want to put patients at risk if he got sloppy and tired, and he really didn't want her overexerting herself and putting her or the baby at risk. He'd told Mack he was only going back to support Jack's return if she was cleared, and his brother had agreed that seemed like a good idea.

Speaking of Mack, he owed his brother a call-back, but it could wait a quick second while he made sure Jack was okay there. His phone buzzed again.

"Everything okay?" she asked. She gestured with her chin to his phone, still gripped tight in his hands.

"Yeah, it's fine. Or maybe not, but I'll handle it in a sec." He went to kiss her and she pulled back.

"I'm not going anywhere, Rhett. And since I'm about to suggest that before we head into work we talk about what has been happening between us, you should handle whatever you need first." She smiled and disrobed, pulling all his focus to the slight swell in her abdomen. He'd never been so happy to see it.

Jack was remarkable. There was no hint of annoyance or frustration in her voice, just the facts. They had time and he needed to get his head right before they dove into the inevitable "what are we" conversation, especially before the gossip mill at work got ahold of them; after all, they'd shown up together in matching ambulances a week ago.

Interestingly, he was looking forward to refuting rumors more than calling Mack back. He and his brother may be making good headway, but they were still brothers. Still just different enough.

"Thanks," he said. Jogging back over to the dresser, he realized his legs were back to normal. Atrophied a bit from lying in bed so much, but overall, he was unscathed. He sent up another prayer of thanks to whomever might be listening. "I'll be right back."

He threw on some sleep pants for now. He'd change when he found out what was expected of him at work.

"You're amazing, by the way," he told Jack.

"You, too, Morrison." She closed the door to the bathroom and he heard the shower start. All he wanted was to join her in it, but she was right—this was important. He'd received more texts from his brother that morning than in the last year combined.

He dialed Mack's number and his brother picked up on the first ring.

"It's about time," he said. There was an urgency behind his brother's cool greeting. Rhett's intuition was heightened.

"Good to hear your voice, too. What's up, Mack? I'm not due at the hospital until six. Unless something is getting in the way of our paperwork to come back?"

"Tyson called in sick with the flu so we're short-staffed. Can you come in early to get checked out? Then if you're cleared, you can stay for a short shift so you don't get worn out."

Rhett appreciated that Mack had already considered the idea for shorter work shifts until they saw how he handled things.

"When do you need me?"

"Like, now?"

Rhett sighed. So much for rest and recuperation. "Yeah. I'll shower and see you in ten."

"Thanks. I owe you. You two doing okay, though?"

Rhett didn't know which version of him and Jack Mack was bringing up—the one that got pummeled by a car or the one making a go of raising a kid together while they navigated a new intimate relationship as well.

"We're fine," he hedged. It was kind of nice that him and Mack were getting more interested in talking to one another, but it still felt foreign.

"Glad to hear it. See you soon."

Rhett hung up and grumbled as he walked into the bathroom. He'd be joining Jack in the shower, but not in the way he'd hoped.

"I've got to head in," he told her. "But mind if I join you?"

"Not at all. Get in here, you." She kissed him, soap sliding down their faces. She laughed and rinsed her hair, her movements slow but smoother than they had been. He was in awe of her quick healing.

He showered quickly, kissed Jack and left, making it to the hospital in less than half an hour from when he talked to Mack. And he hated every minute of being without Jack, of trusting that she could, and would, make it to Austin Memorial safely.

As soon as he walked through the doors, he got a text from his brother.

911. Trauma two. You here?

Good grief. Couldn't he settle in and check the case load before being inundated? He still hadn't even had his final checkup.

Yeah. I'm here. I haven't been cleared, though.

You'll be fine. I'll expedite that if you think you can handle being back?

Could he? He thought so. Heading down.

He moved quickly over to the trauma stations avoiding the looks and whispers from the rest of the staff. He still sported a nice bruise along his cheek from where he'd hit the front passenger seat in the rideshare, not to mention that Austin Memorial was small enough that the rumors had likely gained wings and floated through already. Showing up to work without Jack was probably adding weight to the gossip.

He stopped short at where Mack stood over a patient, performing CPR.

"You're here," Mack said, his voice breaking with emotion. Rhett had mere seconds to recognize that his brother was in crisis. "I—I need your help."

Rhett didn't have time to wonder what his brother meant, or why he was so emotionally distraught. The beeps and trills in the background said the patient was in ventricular fibrillation and losing sinus rhythm. There would be time for questions later.

"How long has he been under?"

"Two minutes. F1 crash at the stadium and he rolled. Likely swelling in his brain. He, uh, he—"

"Hey, I got this," Rhett said. He took over compressions and glanced down at his patient. Sure enough, the guy had pieces of his jumpsuit that hadn't been cut off, showing he was part of the new crew that was training in Austin.

"I thought it was you when they wheeled him in. You weren't answering your phone earlier, and then this—" The admission from his brother made sense on so many levels. The guy did share Rhett's coloring and haircut, though at first glance he was three or four inches shorter than Rhett. It also explained the panic on Mack's face. It was a rarity to see any emotion besides stoic responsibility from his brother; the fear etched on Mack's features scared him. "I know you quit doing the crazy stuff yourself after med school, but it brought it all back after your accident, and now, with a kid of my own on the way—"

"I've got this now, so you can head out and triage what's in the waiting room."

As if hearing his brother's command shocked him out of his own overthinking, Mack shook his head. He cleared his throat, and within seconds, Mack's veneer was back intact like it'd never left.

How long had he kept anything real at bay? This wasn't the time to dive into it, but Rhett and Mack had to have a talk at some point.

"No. I can assist. But take the lead since this is your expertise? I'll be your backup since you just got back."

"You got it."

Rhett worked to get the pressure back online for his patient, then, when he was stable enough not to code in the next thirty seconds, he checked the guy's labs. There was intracranial bleeding and some broken limbs that would obviously take second to the more pressing surgery needed.

"We need to release the pressure," he said. He'd recently watched Jack use a technique with Tanya, the rodeo teen who'd fallen from her horse, that would benefit this patient as well. He made a note to thank her later. A wave of general appreciation for her washed over him, but like talking to Mack, now wasn't the time or place.

"I've called ahead for a room, but they're booked with a multivehicle crash on the 30. This guy won't make it back inside a race car if we don't get an OR in the next few minutes."

Rhett considered their options. Forget racing again; without an immediate decompressive craniectomy, the patient wouldn't live to see the OR to fix the rest of his injuries.

"You feel comfortable doing it here?" Rhett asked Mack.

Mack's lips twisted. "I've done it once, but it wasn't good. You?"

"In the field, but we had a whole team."

"Call in who you need," Mack said. "And let's do it. He doesn't have a chance otherwise."

Rhett nodded and stepped out to rally two nurses who'd just come off the MVC cases. He texted Lainey as well, even though he was pretty sure she was tied up. They could use Jack, but he didn't dare bring her in for this kind of case, not without being 100 percent cleared by a neutral doctor. There was too much at stake with the baby and her own health.

When he got back in the room, Mack and the team had set up a sterile field and closed off the space to anyone else. An anesthesiologist was brought in in case, even though the patient was unconscious. Who knew what would happen when the docs started drilling into his skull.

A flutter of excitement built in Rhett's stomach. He hadn't had a case that made him feel as alive as he had during his time with the rodeo and F1 circuits until now. But was that really a bad thing?

Mack mentioned having a family to take care of now, and for the first time in his life, Rhett understood that on a cellular level. He and Jack might not be a couple in a conventional sense, but they were making a go of raising a kid together. They were sleeping together. He thought of her all the time, at work or otherwise, especially since he'd thought he might lose her.

If he was being honest, he…he *loved* her, and their baby…

That was a rude awakening for a man who tried like hell never to let that happen. But it was true, and he didn't care if he should or shouldn't feel it. Which added a whole level of complication he didn't want to wrestle with at the moment, largely, imagining what it meant to love someone and send them into the world where accidents happened all the time.

He'd thought he'd kept his distance from love so he didn't turn out like his father, but he'd unwittingly also saved himself an immeasurable amount of heartache and potential loss. Now, he either had to accept that risk head-on, or try like hell to shove it back into the depths of his heart from where the feelings originated.

That's impossible. Another truth. He loved Jack and couldn't go back if he tried.

As he shaved the patient's head and taped the gauze around the drill site, Rhett realized something else.

Jack and their unborn child had crossed over into the most important priorities in Rhett's life. Work was something he loved, craved so he knew he was doing good in the world if for no other reason than to offset the awfulness his dad brought.

However, the adventure he craved—the adrenaline and newness every day? Yeah, he got that from being with Jack. And he wanted to protect her at all costs, even if those costs were expensive for him.

Well, hell. What did that mean for him chasing this job? He wanted life on his terms, but those could look different than they did when he'd come to Austin.

Let this go for now. You have a patient. His subconscious was right. Nothing else could matter at the moment. Not Jack, not the baby, not the job could consume his thoughts until his patient was in the clear.

"Okay, let's cut," he said. Mack nodded. "I'm going in anterior and want you ready with the drain."

He and Mack worked in tandem and, though he was worried it was too soon for him to be back at work, especially for a case as intense as this one, he noted how well his brother supported him. They really complemented one another. Mack was precise and efficient to Rhett's quick triage and planning through the surgery. When Rhett seemed tired, Mack picked up the slack, never letting up on the patient's care for a moment.

An excruciating hour later, they laid down

their instruments and took down their masks. The patient wasn't out of the woods yet, but he was going to live long enough to get to the OR when it opened so his bones could be set. There was hope, and in their line of work, sometimes that's all they got.

"That was touch and go but we did it," Rhett said.

"Yeah, we did. And thanks. That hasn't happened before. I mean, me freezing like that."

Rhett patted Mack on the shoulder. It was uncomfortable because physical affection between them was as foreign as talking was. But it was also needed. This was his brother, his family.

"I get it. But I'm okay, and so is Jack."

"You guys scared the hell out of us, that's for sure."

"I know. How are you and Lainey doing?" Rhett asked.

Mack smiled. "I think we're okay. I mean, we're going to have the baby we always wanted and we're doing the work we were too immature to do the first time around. It's kind of…perfect. I want the same for you." Mack didn't add "and Jack," but maybe that was intentional. Rhett hadn't shared his newly discovered feelings.

"Forgive me if I'm overstepping, but there's never really been anyone else for you, right? How… How'd you know?"

Mack shook his head and stared at the tablet. "No. There hasn't been. It's…it's always been Lainey." Rhett had a million questions for his brother, but Mack patted him on the shoulder. "Actually, I should go. Do you mind finishing up here? I mean, do you think you're okay to?"

"Not at all," Rhett said. "Go, and I can finish up. This is the easy stuff."

"Thanks. I'm sorry, I just have something to do that can't wait." Mack handed over the tablet with the patient's chart and headed toward the door.

"Of course. And, Mack?"

Mack's head turned. "Thanks. It was nice working with you." There was more he wanted to say but none of it mattered in the moment. He was grateful they'd finally had a chance to spend time with one another, that they were working through their childhood issues and coming together over medicine at least.

They had a ways to go, but they were making steady ground. The accident was scary as hell, but maybe it served a bigger purpose after all.

To add to that, Mack was being brave. He was showing up for his family where and when he was needed. Maybe it wasn't too late; Rhett could learn a thing or two from his older brother.

Once the chart was updated and the F1 patient was transferred to ortho for his other injuries, Rhett made his way to the cafeteria to grab a coffee and sit for a moment. His legs shook with the exertion of being on his feet for a few hours for the first time in days.

He also needed to decompress and think through the last few hours. First, he pulled out his phone to make sure he didn't have any pressing needs to attend to first.

Only two. Not bad. The first was an email marked "Urgent" and the second, a text from Jack. The latter made him smile, and since he wanted to carry that into the rest of his day, he checked the email first.

Everett, it began.

A birdie at Austin Memorial told me you're working there now. Good for you. I know Mack wanted to connect with you at some point and talk to you about a job. This seems like a good fit.

However, the reason I'm reaching out is because the same birdie told me you're on your way to fatherhood. Congratulations, Everett. There's no greater gift than seeing your family expand and watch as your children surpass you.

To that end, I'm writing to see when I can meet the lucky lady you chose to start a family with. I know you and I haven't always been close, but seeing as how you have met the terms of the inheritance, with one exception, I'm hoping we can work past our differences so I can be a part of your growing family.

That, in case you don't recall, is the last part of the clause for the trust to be released to you: I get to have the opportunity to be involved in yours and your family's lives. It's a big ask, I know, but I'm willing to pay for it, enough that you won't have to worry about the costs of raising a child in today's economy, or worry about giving them the best life possible.

All I need in return is a second chance. Mack is on board, let me know if you are as well. Give it some thought and get back to me, son.

Dad

Rhett's hands shook. There were so many triggers in that email he could barely track them all. To start, his father wanted a second chance? If Everett were stupid enough to let him back in, it would be way more than a second chance. Try fourteenth. Twentieth. Hundredth, depending on what one considered a "chance" at earning his son's trust.

And then he'd dared to add the addendum that he had to have a relationship with whomever Rhett had impregnated. An innocent bystander who didn't deserve to be brought into Morrison family drama.

Nothing about the accident, nothing about

wanting to repair the damage from their past. No apology for being absent most of Rhett's life. Nothing real. Just his dad issuing more demands.

It was unconscionable.

Rhett was already against accessing the trust fund, feeling like it was a seedy way to get Morrison blood to propagate. But this made it sleazy. Thom was trying to buy favor with his sons, who he'd perpetually disappointed their whole lives. No, that wasn't even the worst part. Thom hadn't even asked about Rhett's partner, just said he wanted to meet her and was "willing to pay for it."

Gross.

How, in good conscience, could Rhett agree? His dad had said Mack was "on board," but there was no way that was true. More than likely it was another hook designed to get Rhett to think he was the outlier, the one keeping their family from connecting. It was par for the course, then.

Either way, that talk with his brother needed to happen sooner rather than later, it seemed. Mack deserved to know what their dad was up to, especially when he'd worked as hard as he had to keep the man from his life as well.

He flipped off the phone until he recalled he had a text from Jack. He took a deep, calming breath in and opened it. It turned out there were three texts.

Hey, you! I am approved to go back to work! Mack has me working on a case that has me off my feet (of course, since he's—what did you call it? An "overprotective ass"?), but I thought when I'm done, we could grab some dinner? Call me crazy but we might have a thing or two to still talk about, haha.

That was an understatement. He kept reading.

Oh, and I'm buying dinner as a way to say thank you for the apartment and willingness to explore whatever this might be; I know it's a lot for you to take on, me and the baby, when you weren't sure you wanted either in the beginning.

He didn't deserve the thanks, not especially because she was right; he hadn't been sure about her, not really until he thought he'd lose her. What kind of a man did that make him? And would he revert right back to the guy he'd been before once things settled—a man who put himself first so he could avoid any complications that might be too similar to how he was raised?

And there was another concern that had cropped up with that email. Would he be forced to say goodbye to her in order to keep her from his father?

On that note, I really enjoyed our "exploration" this morning and hope there's more to come as we both heal. It'll make raising this kiddo together a whole lot more fun. ;) Anyway, hope to see you at dinner.

Rhett's deep breath, and all the oxygen it was supposed to supply his blood, was completely ineffective. He felt like a two-hundred-pound anvil was sitting on top of his chest. Getting air was impossible, and his head was spinning.

Was he having a heart attack?

He fumbled his way to a seat in the back of the cafeteria and put his head between his legs. If there was a blood clot they'd missed when he was here after the accident… But no, with his head bent over, it was a little easier to draw a breath, and his pulse slowed. It was probably just a panic attack, but that wasn't good, either, not with what he'd chosen as his profession.

The next question, now that he had enough oxygen to his brain to think clearly, was to find out why he was feeling this way. It was about Jack, obviously. And the email from his dad. But why did he let the email get to him at all? Why not just tell his dad to shove off and that he didn't want the trust? That was the plan all along, wasn't it?

Because secretly, you do want a relationship with your dad, just not the one you've grown up with. You're afraid if you say yes to this deal, as he claimed Mack has, you'll let him back in and he'll disappoint you, again. Then, you'll be exactly where you are now, with nothing but more bad memories to flood your system. Those will affect your new family.

Then he should say no.

Yeah, like it's that easy. If the offer is always out there, you'll always wonder.

So, what *was* the answer?

Before he could overthink it, he wrote out a reply to his father. Maybe he should talk to Mack first, maybe even involve Jack, but neither would help him through these complicated emotions around his relationship with his dad.

Dad, thank you for the offer, but I'll have to respectfully decline. The woman and I, unlike Mack and Lainey, aren't together. The pregnancy was a mistake and we will need to find our way through co-parenting before we involve anyone else in this mess we created. Thank you, though. Be well.

Again, his hands shook as he hit Send. There. It was done. It wasn't necessarily true, but it wasn't a lie, either. He and Jack weren't together, not really, and the pregnancy was an accident, if not a mistake, though he'd never allow himself to believe the latter. As long as his father believed what he'd written, that was all that mattered.

It wasn't as if the man ever came to Austin or reached out to chat with his sons. How would he really know if Jack and him were spending time together or not?

He wasn't sure how he was going to answer her when she asked him how he felt at dinner, but at least this mess was behind him. They could keep figuring out who and what they were, without the prying eyes of whoever the "little birdie" was. If it was Mack, though…

Anger rolled through him, hot and liquid. No. They'd made too much progress for Mack to steamroll him like that.

His phone chimed again.

Jack. He smiled like he did every time he saw her name on his screen and flipped the phone open.

I didn't know you felt that way, but I'm glad to hear you being honest again. Obviously, we don't need to grab dinner, but we should still probably talk, this time about whether you want me to move out or not. Now that I'm healthy, that shouldn't be a problem. Sorry for being an inconvenience.

Rhett was confused. What did she mean "move out"? they'd had an amazing morning together, connecting and sharing intimacy that made Rhett's toes curl to recall. Then he'd come into work, talked to Mack, gotten the email from his dad—

Oh, no. The email. He opened it again, checking the "To" line, like he should have earlier. Sure enough, there was another email address listed.

J.Elliot@austinmemorial.org.

Damn, damn, damn.

His duplicitous, self-serving old man had found Jack's email address and included her in the missive that was both offensive and toxic—more so now that he knew Jack had read it.

Worse? She'd assumed he meant every word of it, and why wouldn't she? It was his voice, and he was the one putting off the "what are we" conversation.

He put his phone away and tore off in the direction of his brother's office. Yes, he needed to ask his brother more than a few pointed questions, but he also had to find out where Mack had Jack working the next few days so Rhett could fix this huge mistake before it blew up in his face. He just needed to stall until he figured out what he could say to make this right. He'd only get one chance to fix this, of that he was certain.

Please, he whispered, *please let me figure out what I need to say to her before it's too late.*

CHAPTER TEN

JACK'S HANDS FIDDLED with the puzzle pieces, picking them apart and putting them in the appropriate boxes. It was a benign activity that had nothing to do with medicine, but that was the premise of her "task" from Mack.

She was supposed to put together puzzles with one of the peds in the long-term care unit at Austin M, searching for any signs of the palsy returning to the young girl's dexterity. Katie, an eleven year old with a penchant for boy bands and mint chocolate-chip ice cream, had a resection of a brain tumor a few months prior, and her parents had just gotten ready to bring her home when the tremors from a compressed nerve returned.

The scans showed that Katie had a recurrence of the tumor, and it had grown quickly. The problem was, the palsy caused as a result of the tumor was making it difficult to get the tumor completely resected. If they cut now, while she was having seizures every few minutes, the likelihood of a negative outcome in surgery went through the roof. It was old-fashioned to do it this way, but it was so much more low-risk for the patient when she was relaxed doing puzzles than tied up to wires and machines.

Jack tried to concentrate on the puzzle they'd moved on to, but she'd had two strange experiences back-to-back. First, the day before, Lainey had found her and told her that she and Mack were engaged! They were going to have a small private wedding and Jack, for one, couldn't be happier. Sure, a small hint of jealousy had cropped up, but how could she be anything other than thrilled that her friend had gotten back together with her husband, especially since they were expecting a child together?

The second, less amazing news caused the jealousy for Lainey and Mack's impending nuptials to skyrocket, though. It also made her nauseated enough she ran to the bathroom and lost what was left of her breakfast.

In an email to his father that she was copied in on, Rhett had said that he wasn't with her, that their baby was a mistake and that she was no more than a woman he'd knocked up. And then he'd worked all night, leaving her alone with her thoughts.

"Dr. Elliot?" Katie asked. "Do you have any corner pieces?"

Jack nodded and smiled, though it felt forced.

She focused on the girl's hand as she handed over the corner pieces she'd culled. Sure enough, the tremor was there, and more pronounced than earlier. She made a note of it and chatted with Katie for a bit before they went back to working in silence.

Just like that, the email slipped back in. All she could think about were the words Rhett had written back to his father. Sure, the original email from Thom Morrison had been a little strange with all the discussion of trusts and language she'd never spoken in her life, but Rhett's dad seemed nice enough.

Which was why the email response from Rhett didn't make sense. She'd read it multiple times, hoping there was a clue that he hadn't meant it, that his callousness wasn't real. Maybe he hadn't seen her on the email chain, but all that meant was he thought she wouldn't see it. And then to come home and sleep on the couch so he could work on charts all night? To use work as an excuse instead of facing the fire with her?

She was confused, hurt and felt…betrayed. She'd really thought they had something.

"Dr. Elliot, there's a cute doctor out there," Katie said.

Jack laughed and handed Katie some edge pieces to the beach puzzle they were working on.

"Oh yeah? We've got a few of those on this

floor, don't we?" Only one came to mind for her, though, and he was a trauma doc. Ugh. Why couldn't she put Rhett from her mind? "Aren't you a little young to be checking out doctors, Katie?" She watched the girl's hands again. The tremor persisted. *Hmm.* In other circumstances the puzzle would be relaxing, but not while she needed to track a poor girl's tumor and its devastating effects.

How would Jack react if anything like this happened to her daughter? Katie's parents must be a wreck not being able to be there every day; they both had to work to keep the health insurance that guaranteed they wouldn't go completely bankrupt caring for Katie, so they only came in the evenings to play cards and watch a movie with their daughter. Over the past two weeks, Jack had seen them look more and more exhausted, and she didn't blame them one bit. But they were a couple, and drew on each other for strength. It was clear Jack wouldn't have that.

"I'm not too young. My best friend already has a boyfriend that sends her candy to her class." Jack stifled a laugh when she saw the earnestness on the girl's face. "Besides, this one's the cutest. And I haven't seen him before."

Jack turned around, and sure enough, Rhett stood in the doorway, an easy smile on his face while he watched Jack pick through cerulean and beige puzzle pieces with Katie.

“Hi there, ladies. How’s it going in here?”

“We’re great!” Katie exclaimed, at the same time Jack said, “Fine.” Katie sat up straighter and fluffed her hair. Jack made a mental note to bring some clips in the next day to do Katie’s hair for her.

“I’m Dr. Morrison and I work downstairs in the ER.”

“I’m Katie, and this is Dr. Elliot. We’re building puzzles and looking for my palsy shakes. I didn’t know there were two Dr. Morrisons.”

Jack winced. The girl knew so much about what was going on with her and was still so brave. Maybe Jack could be, too.

“The other Dr. Morrison is my brother, and he’s in charge of a lot of other doctors. I know Dr. Elliot. She and I work together.”

“Dr. Elliot, they’re both cute!” Katie hissed. Jack assumed the girl meant both Morrison brothers. She didn’t disagree, but only one had her heart.

“Katie, do you mind if I talk to Dr. Elliot in the hallway really quick?”

Katie nodded exuberantly even though she had no idea what the two doctors were going to talk about. Namely, what an idiot Jack had been for trusting that Rhett really cared about her when he'd never actually articulated that. Sure, he'd been comfortable hooking up with her, even living with her because it kept things easy. But when it came to caring, he'd never said a word to her.

"Sure, Dr. Morrison. Take all the time you need." Katie gave Jack an exaggerated wink. Oh boy. That girl would be trouble when she got out of here and hit her teenage years.

If she got out. Jack's hand rested on her belly. Parenting was the scariest thing there was, wasn't it? The only thing second to it was putting her heart on the line one more time.

She followed Rhett into the hallway and channeled Katie's bravery.

"What are you doing here, Rhett? I made it clear I got your message and when I called off dinner and slept on the couch, I hoped you realized that talking about this isn't necessary. Nor is checking up on me anymore."

Rhett didn't go to her, didn't move in her direction, but his face wore the same expression as when they made love and his gaze connected with hers. Gosh, she wished she didn't know exactly what that looked like, felt like, sounded like when he whispered into her ear as they climaxed together.

"I'm sorry I had to fill charts, or that I chose to. To be honest, I was trying to head off talking until I knew what to say. I also know what you think you read, but can I talk to you about it now that I have a handle on things? Will you hear me out?"

She nodded and he exhaled, moving a foot closer to her. She fought the urge to run backward where his scent and presence couldn't trick her again. She didn't owe him anything, but the magnetic pull was too much.

"You have five minutes, then I'm back to puzzle-making with Katie."

"I won't need that long, hopefully. For starters, I'm deeply sorry you saw that, but not that I wrote it." The look on her face must have registered her surprise because he waved her off. "Let me explain. My dad and I have a complicated relationship, Jack. In the interest of time, seeing as how I'm down to four minutes, I'll give you the abridged version, some of which you know. He cheated on my mom with a dozen other women that we know of, fathering at least one sister we only sort of know. He ruined our lives and my mom got sick, but didn't have the energy to fight it, so she died, leaving us with him and no real role model. Mack, as you know, went one way to stave off what we call the Morrison curse, and I went the other. I'd like to think we're meeting in the middle now."

"Me, too," she added. They did seem to be closer than ever before. Both seemed…different. Better, stronger, more nuanced. She felt the same about herself, but then, she was growing a human, so of course she was different.

"Anyway, I am sorry again that you saw my message back to him, but it was the only way to shake him off. If he feels like he has an in, he'll exploit it till he ruins everything in his path. I won't let him get close to you or our little bean, even if it means lying to him to get him off our scent."

He'd ended up in front of her, and she wanted to melt into him. It'd been over a day since she'd left the bed with him in it, and she missed him deeply. What was she supposed to do, other than believe him? She sat in silence for thirty seconds, mulling her feelings and options. She loved the man and searched her heart for hints he might be lying to her, or trying to manipulate the situation.

She found none, but still had some questions.

"Can we talk, then, about where we are?"

"We're here, together, at least in my opinion."

"How so? Because combined with this email to your dad, the way you've pushed off this conversation means the evidence points to you not wanting to be with me. That leaves us less to talk about."

He seemed to consider that, as did a few peds nurses who giggled when they walked by him. Apparently, he was a hot item to more than just the peds patients. Go figure.

"I like you, Jack." He paused and not for the first time, she wished she had access to what he was thinking in the silence. "A lot. And I want to be with you in any way that I can. Right now, that means showing up for you and this baby we created and making sure you're safe and cared for."

"You don't think it's a mistake? The baby? I know you didn't want kids at all when I met you."

Rhett chuckled. "I didn't, and I'm still not sure I'll be a good dad. But I'll do my best and no, this isn't a mistake at all. No matter how it happened, it's a miracle, and I'm glad to be doing it with you."

"That's all I can ask for. So, to be clear, for you and I, we're…"

"Living and raising a baby together and hopefully working toward doing that while we get to know one another more. I don't have a label for it, and I know you want one, but this is all I have for now. I know I care about you so much, and that's something I'm not used to. I'd like to explore that if you're up for taking it slowly. I also enjoy working with you more than you know."

She understood. Sort of.

It was more than she expected, but was it enough to build a life around? It had to be, for now at least.

"Okay. I'll do my best. But so you know, your brother may have let it slip that a permanent position at the clinic could be opening up and that's what my heart is set on doing."

"I hadn't heard that, but I agree, you'd be the best fit by a long shot. I'll miss you here, but I'll help in any way I can."

"Thank you, Rhett. I'm going to go for it, but I'm also going to keep my name in here because I can't put all my eggs in this basket if the job at the clinic doesn't work out, and you don't know what you want, Rhett. Please don't take it personally, but I've had enough of life lived outside my control. I need to take care of myself and our child first."

A shadow fell on his face, but he managed to keep his gentle smile. "I wouldn't expect anything less. I hope you get it, to be honest. You're so good with these little guys. Austin Memorial would be lucky to have you."

"Thanks. Speaking of, I should get back to Katie. If she finishes that puzzle without me, I'll never hear the end of it."

"Will I see you at home?" he asked. The shadow had passed but his smile was weak. "I'd like to have that dinner with you to celebrate both of us being healthy enough to be back at work."

Rhett might not know what he wanted long-term, but he said all the right things most of the time. It was confusing, but she could be patient. After all, they had seven more months to figure out how to co-parent, seven more months to see who got the job and who had to find other arrangements. Seven months to hope Rhett figured out what he wanted.

So long as she could still live with Rhett if she didn't get the position, she would be okay. Hopefully the clinic panned out so she could have something not just permanent, but fulfilling.

So much weighed was on her mind as she went back to Katie's room, but no sooner was she inside than she blanched.

"Dr. Morrison!" she cried. Rhett came running back in the room, his gait still stunted from their accident. "She's seizing. Help me stabilize her?"

"Of course. Where do you want me?"

"She's better on her right side, so can you roll her toward me?" Normally that wouldn't be a question she'd ask; Rhett was stronger than most athletes she'd met. But the accident had weakened both of them. They had to administer her medication, but it was nearly impossible, even with the port for her IV. Katie hadn't had a seizure this strong since she was admitted.

"Does this happen often, or was it just the palsy?"

"This is abnormal for sure," Jack said. She got the meds in and still, nothing. "Dammit. She's not responding."

"Do you think the tumor is impeding her nerves

in a new way, or that her brain is decompensating with the stress? That'll change the reaction to the meds."

"Agreed. We need to wheel her down to get another scan when she's stable. This is bad."

He nodded. "Are you sure you're up for it? This kind of stress on your body—"

"I'll be fine if you're with me."

"I'm not going anywhere until you tell me to. I'm yours."

It was so easy for Rhett to make that promise to her where work was concerned, that she could almost believe he meant it outside the hospital as well. Jack tucked it away, wishing it were true. How much more could she accomplish when she was supported with that kind of certainty?

Together, they were a fully operating unit, and in that moment, she was thankful for the assistance. After nearly three minutes, Katie moved out of the seizure, but she was still unconscious.

In the elevator, Jack's hand rested on her stomach. Were they crazy to bring a child into a world with so much uncertainty? Not just with the world at large—though that was wild enough. Look at Rhett's career of caring for people hurt doing what they loved. She'd balked at that kind of risk, but then he was right, wasn't he? The risk was there either way, just by existing. To think any of them could avoid it was so naive, so silly, it almost buckled her at the knees.

A small cry escaped her lips, a release of some of the heavy emotions she'd kept bottled up inside her for months now while she escaped the horror of her old life and worked like hell to begin a new one.

Rhett took her hand as they waited to make it to the third floor where the CT and imaging was.

"She'll be okay."

"I know. Katie's a trooper." She sniffled, making herself believe it, or what were they doing there?

Rhett squeezed her hand. "I mean our little bean. I know you're scared, but no matter what happens to us, she'll be alright."

Jack had to believe that, too. She had to imagine a world where a loved child, even with parents who cared about one another but were at odds with their storied pasts, could thrive.

Or, again, what would be the point of it all?

The elevator doors opened and they wheeled Katie to the imaging center. Jack tucked her own worry away, knowing it would be there once this crisis was averted. That was the similarity between being a doctor and a parent, wasn't it? Both required you to put aside your own fears and joys to take care of someone else's.

She could do that, but at what point would she

break under all that pressure, especially as she faced it alone? She hoped she didn't have to find out, but the nerves turning her stomach told her avoiding a breakdown might not be in her cards.

If that was true, she hoped she at least had someplace safe to land when it happened. With that, she focused everything on saving the little girl in front of her.

This is all I can control right now. And that has to be enough.

In her heart, though, she knew it wasn't. Too bad there wasn't a thing she could do about it.

CHAPTER ELEVEN

RHETT LEFT THE peds wing feeling like his world was off-kilter. Jack was the strongest woman he knew, and she was braving so much. Leaving an abusive husband, starting a new life where she relied only on herself, finding out she was pregnant with the man who she was fighting for a job…

All she asked for was certainty from him and he couldn't give it. What the actual hell was wrong with him? He'd been so sure after the accident that he loved her, and that hadn't changed. They were still sleeping together, still supporting one another, still planning to raise a baby together.

He'd taken a night to be sure he was ready to have that conversation she kept asking for, was pretty sure they were on the same page. Or at least they had been…

So, what changed?

My dad's email. That had to be it.

But he'd squashed that, hadn't he? Sort of. He'd said his piece, but was that handling it, or pushing the crisis to a later date so he didn't have to cope with it now? The way he'd brushed off her question about what they were didn't sit well with him.

You're letting him get to you, even if you think you're being different. Are you, really? I mean, you're having a baby and won't even commit.

Shit. Is that what he was doing?

All he knew was that he wanted to be there for Jack, but something tethered him to his old ways. His dad or something else, he couldn't definitively say. Until he figured it out and put it to rest for good, he'd be stuck here.

And how patient could she expect to be? He didn't want to find out.

At the same time, he wasn't ready to go home and have her ask him what they were, which meant he was in the same position as the night before. He didn't know, and any attempt at this point to work through his feelings in front of her would only make things worse.

Rhett worked the rest of his short shift, which brought him into that evening feeling depleted and like he'd gone twenty rounds with a prizefighter. The only thing that got him through was imagining how good it would feel to go home, take Jack in his arms and tell her he'd gotten it all wrong. It seemed so easy when he pictured it.

But was he able to do that? Really?

Sure, he felt that way, but he was also confused. If he did, why were the words still stuck in his throat? Luckily, the work had come to him easy, the traumas coming through a welcome distraction from watching his own heart bleeding out on the table that was his life.

Only one case gave him pause, a thirty-week pregnant woman who'd sustained blunt trauma to her abdomen and cerebral spine, courtesy of an intoxicated driver. She didn't look like Jack, save their obvious shared condition, but seeing the woman lifeless on the gurney, two lives at stake, almost did him in.

Thankfully, Mack came in and took over, pretending to need Rhett in another case where an older gentleman had fallen from a ladder trying to take down his son-in-law's Christmas lights in April.

He'd crossed paths with Jack twice in the first half of her second shift back, but then she'd gone home like he should have if he weren't punishing his body so his mind would quiet. She'd barely glanced at him, and he wondered if she was thinking, as he was, of his paltry reply to what she had asked about their relationship.

His body craved hers, and when she was in his arms he felt like home. Missing her the night before had showed him how empty his life was without her in it. That should be all that mattered.

Do the work. Fix your shit and find a way past your past.

Sure. Like it was that easy.

If he made the commitment to her and he couldn't honor it—for whatever reason, especially the unnamed one holding him back right now—he'd only hurt her worse down the line.

So tell her that.

No. How could he tell a woman he cared for, who was pregnant with his baby, that he didn't know if he could give her what she wanted? He'd opened a line of emotional credit with her and was running up his interest with no plan to pay her back.

Needs, not wants. She wants a hot cup of tea and milk each night, preferably with a chocolate biscuit, but she needs and deserves a man who can put aside his neuroses and show up for her when it counts.

She texted, asking when he'd be home, that she was getting sleepy but still wanted to talk. She'd wait for dinner, but was just going to have a snack to make sure the baby got what she needed.

Why don't you get some rest and we can tackle this tomorrow, he replied. I'm still working here anyway, so go ahead with dinner.

Technically that wasn't true—his shift was over and he could go home at any time. But he couldn't. Not with so much on his mind and heart; he couldn't bring that home to her. He'd tried the night before and hadn't been able to cross the threshold of their bedroom. Was this worse? Maybe, but surely not as bad as letting her down by not being ready.

Sure. Fine. Have a good night.

He knew he was avoiding her. Avoiding a serious conversation that would hold his feet to the fire. Maybe that made him a coward, but if he pushed it off, he didn't run the risk of losing her, and that had to be enough for now.

His phone buzzed again, and he swiped it open without glancing at the home screen.

It was just Mack, asking to see him in his office. Rhett needed to calm the hell down; he still worried without Jack by his side that there would be a complication, that she'd be showing up on a gurney at Austin M.

"I'll be by before I leave," he said in a voice text reply.

He swung by Human Resources first, to find out if there were any other openings he could apply for. He didn't care if he worked at the new trauma clinic or hell, even the birthing center. He just wanted to take one thing off Jack's plate that was within his control—without damning himself in the process. Because he could leave Austin Memorial and make it easy on her, but selfishly, leaving her was an impossibility.

"'Fraid not," the woman at the desk told him.

"They pulled the job announcements when we got the extra funding. Apparently they have people slated for them. Sorry."

"That's okay. Thanks for checking." He was mildly annoyed that Mack was sticking to his guns to hire from outside the building to make sure they had coverage in the ER at the main Austin M location. They had too many people for the ER, if Rhett and Jack were still vying for the same position.

He got pulled back into two more cases before he remembered he was supposed to go see Mack. The guy wasn't in his office, though, so Rhett figured he'd text when he got home.

Almost a full five hours later, he was on his way out the door, when he saw Mack in his periphery. He was talking to someone whose back faced Rhett, but he still seemed familiar. When they shook hands and the man clapped Mack on the back before he walked away, Rhett froze.

Surely his eyes were tired from the interminable shift he'd just worked. He had to be seeing things because if he wasn't, there was a problem.

He blinked, rubbed his dry eyes, and sure as hell, he knew the guy.

Their father. What was he doing there? He was out the door before Rhett could ask him, though.

Mack's smile—a rarity as it was—fell when he saw Rhett.

"What the hell are you doing bringing him here?" Rhett hissed.

"Let's talk in my office. There've been some developments."

"I need some sleep, Mack. I just pulled a twelve on my first day back, and I'm wiped. But before I go, I need to know what the hell our dad was doing in our hospital."

Mack held out his arm, gesturing to the elevator. "Come talk to me. You'll want to hear this, I promise."

Somehow, Rhett didn't think that was true. He shot Jack a text that he'd be home soon and would cook her a meal she'd never forget when she woke up. At least, he could give her that. Right away, the three blinking dots came on the screen saying she was replying, but they vanished and nothing appeared.

Why was she awake? Was she okay?

She's fine, he assured himself. Just probably overstimulated from her first day at work. Still, worry settled deep in his stomach.

"I want to take the stairs. Good to get the blood flowing." Mack nodded his agreement.

"How'd the patient do?" he asked Mack. "The pregnant one?" He needed to change the subject, think about anything other than his father.

Mack's jaw hardened. "The baby is fine, but

will need to be in the NICU for a while. There were too many complications."

Rhett understood what his brother wouldn't say. The worry in his stomach turned to stone. Life could shift on a dime, as evidenced by his own accident. Time was one more thing out of his control, as was keeping Jack safe.

All he could do was be there for her and hope it was enough.

See? That's all commitment is—making that choice every day.

He could do that. One of many locks around his heart clicked open. There were a few still to go, but he was making progress.

"I'm so sorry to hear that. The husband must be gutted."

"He is. They'd been trying for years to have a kid and now he has to raise her himself."

"That's awful. Makes you think, doesn't it?"

"It does," his brother said. They both understood on a very real level what was at stake in their own lives. Rhett was deeply grateful in that moment to have his brother in his corner. For that, at least. There was still the unspoken question about what Mack was doing talking to the one man they both swore they wanted out of their life.

He made it to Mack's office on the second floor winded and frustrated. Trying to take the stairs as part of his physical therapy was good in theory, but racing up them with the intent to give his brother a piece of his mind wasn't smart. Especially after finding out his patient had died. What a mess.

Mack walked into his office without waiting for Rhett.

"Well, come on in."

"You're the one who called me up here. What's up?"

"Well, I'll start with the really good news."

Rhett didn't want to know if what followed was more "good" news, or bad news. With their dad involved, it could only be the latter, but Rhett gave Mack the benefit of the doubt.

"Shoot."

"Lainey and I are getting remarried."

Rhett couldn't contain his smile. Before he could overthink it, he hugged Mack tight. "Congratulations. This *is* really good news. When?"

"As soon as the woman will have me. I'm not messing this up again."

Rhett let that sink in. "Can I ask you something?" Mack gestured that he continue. "How did you know you were ready to make that leap? I mean, you and I aren't exactly batting a thousand when it comes to relationships."

"That's part of what you saw with Dad." Rhett frowned, but Mack shook his head. "I know your feelings about him, but he's trying this time. That doesn't mean I'm letting him in the inner sanctum—"

"You have an inner sanctum?" Mack had always struck him as a lone wolf.

"Yeah, smart-ass. You, Lainey, and even Jack. You three are family in a way our old man never was. That said, he's written a couple times and reached out in a way that makes sense to me. I know my boundaries when it comes to him, but so far, he's held that line." He paused. "Also, he's sick. I don't want him to hang out every day, but I would like my kid to know his grandfather."

Rhett felt as if Mack had walked up to him and punched him in the gut. The wind was completely knocked out of him.

"Cancer?" Mack nodded. "Shit." A lifetime of regret filled his lungs, replacing the oxygen. It was hard to breathe with the news—both what he'd expected and not received from his old man and what he should have done sooner to get to where Mack was with him.

"Yeah."

"He here for treatment?"

"Part of that, yes. The rest is part of his agreement with me and Austin Memorial."

Rhett bristled. "You're gonna need to tell me more than that. We can talk about his prognosis later, but if you have an agreement, I need to know."

Mack assessed him through his typical stoic gaze.

"Tell me more about what you meant three weeks ago when I gave you and Dr. Elliot your schedules for the temporary postings."

"What do you mean? What's that got to do with Dad?"

"Just answer. I want to know what you discovered when you told me you'd need to see if this place had the ability to give you more. Does it?"

Everett was sick of the condescension from Mack. "I said I wanted to know if it could give me what I needed."

"Right. Well, does it?"

"I don't know what you mean, specifically, Mack. Can you stop being so clinical and just ask the question you want to ask? You want to know if I am going to leave, right?"

His frustration was back in full force. Here they went again, Rhett being chastised by his bigger brother.

"I mean I don't know where you're coming from." Rhett opened his mouth to say that yeah, Mack damn well did because when they had their annual fundraisers for respective jobs, Mack was always quick to make a comment about Everett's "irresponsible choices" with respect to his career.

Sure, he hadn't done that since he'd been in Austin, but the lingering effects were still there. "And before you chime in with a quick quip about coming from your time as a trauma medic on the circuit, that's not what I mean. I want to know what you felt you were missing that Austin Memorial can give you. I want to know what you think you need right now and if those needs are being met. And I don't mean a paycheck or steady job, Rhett. I want to know if this is the kind of medicine that fulfills you, if this team supports you."

Rhett's chest compressed. This was…*new*. He and his brother didn't talk, certainly not about the things that mattered most to both of them. They were just too different. But they were on the verge of something serious, and damn if it didn't make Rhett want to run for the hills.

If you want different results, you have to do things differently.

Which meant sitting in discomfort and just… listening. Fuck, this was harder than he thought. But another lock clicked open as he allowed that to happen. He just sat and felt the discomfort instead of moving to distract himself or lessen it.

"Let me share something with you, then you can chime in." Rhett nodded and Mack continued. "I'm sorry about the grief I've given you the past few years." Rhett's brows raised as if to say "few?" But at the same time, his pulse quickened. Where was this coming from? "Okay, yeah, maybe more than a few. Anyway, I saw you making what I assumed was mistake after mistake with your career and couldn't understand why you'd want to keep uprooting yourself because that's what Dad did. You and I always swore we'd never live like him."

"I was taking those jobs because I didn't want to get bored and stagnant and then take it out on everyone around me. Dad took on women and it ruined us. Jobs were controllable and didn't affect anyone but me."

"I know. And I know I went about things differently, but we both went about them wrong." And there it was; his brother was passing judgment on Rhett's life again. "We assumed that by keeping love and stability in that way from our lives we wouldn't end up like Dad, but the truth is, we were turning out just like him because we refused to turn into ourselves and do what needed to be done for the people we care about."

Rhett's heart thumped in time with the truth.

"Where is this coming from?"

"Dad and I very recently reconnected, and I know he wants to do that with you. You should hear him out, Rhett. He's done a lot of work, or at least enough it's worth seeing if you still feel the same or you're both different enough to try and forge a new kind of relationship."

Rhett's skin felt like it was being scraped off he was so uncomfortable.

"What is his deal with the hospital?" he asked. He didn't want to think about his brother's suggestion, especially knowing their old man was sick. He didn't want to think about how he'd been wondering the same thing—whether he should just rip the Band-Aid and see what festering wound was underneath or if it had, in fact healed. But the unknown was painful to even think about.

If his father was still a jerk, then he'd be justified in his anger held on to all these years. If not, it meant Rhett had wasted who knew how long being upset for no reason. He didn't know if he could live with himself if that was the truth facing him on the other end of his own nose.

"That depends. Does this place, does practicing this type of medicine fulfill you? Could you really stay and build a life here in our community? Because if you can, I'd like to officially offer you the trauma position."

"Seriously? Just like that?"

"Well, not just like that. How do you feel about Austin Memorial? About working with me?"

Had Mack asked that a month ago, it would have been easy to answer—Rhett wouldn't have been able to handle what felt like stagnation after a lifetime of chasing chaos. Working for Mack would have been okay as a stepping stone, but he'd have wanted his own life. But now he knew differently.

"I love the intensity and kind of cases we see here, don't get me wrong, but I can find that anywhere." The truth bubbled below the surface, aching to get out. Mack's face was expressionless as he waited for Rhett to continue. "But I want to stay because you're right. Being part of a community feels better than I thought it would. I don't want to disappoint them, or you, or myself by looking for more."

Then why can't you just tell that to Jack?

Because she deserved more from him than the kind of commitment he gave to his job. She deserved to know he'd support her through everything that came down their path and he couldn't promise that, not without knowing more about his dad, and about his own hang-ups there.

"I'm glad to hear that. I feel the same. For what it's worth, I'd be proud of you no matter what you chose to do about Austin Memorial. You're doing good things, Rhett."

Another lock clicked open. That made three, but how many more were dead-bolted tight? At least a couple…

"What does this have to do with Dad?" he asked. That particular unknown still plagued him.

"He's donated a substantial sum of money—my part of the inheritance I told him I no longer would accept—to enhancing our birthing center and taking on qualified staff for at least a five-year contract." Rhett's brows raised in question. Their dad was funding the hospital? It made it a little hard to make amends when the guy was, again, hoping he could buy it instead of earning it. "And yeah, I know it seems like nepotism fueled by guilt, but he's doing the best he can and you have a job. Just appreciate that."

Rhett scoffed, rolling back his shoulders and cracking his knuckles. His whole body felt like it was on fire.

"You know damn good and well how much it effing matters. If Dad is puppeteering things here, these jobs aren't stable. He can pull the funding anytime he wants."

Mack sighed and shook his head. "He can't pull the funding. I've had the hospital lawyers look at the contract and the money is Austin Memorial's, no strings attached. I think we might want to admit this is Dad doing a good thing, finally."

Rhett got up and paced. "He's doing this 'good thing' because we turned down the inheritances."

"I know," Mack said. "At least this allows us to open up medical facilities to people who need it, people like Jack and Lainey. He's using his money for good, and he's dropped the talk about being involved in our lives if he does this. He's going about it naturally."

Rhett's skin felt itchy, and his lungs like he couldn't draw in a deep enough breath. "If we let him do this, we're beholden to him forever."

"We're not, Rhett. Can't you see that? You get to make those choices. You can talk to him or not, but the money has been allocated. If I didn't tell you, you wouldn't even know where the funding came from. To be honest, who knows where Dad will be in two years—"

"Don't. Not with the guilt, please, Mack," Rhett sighed and the claustrophobia set in. He should be home, talking to Jack, but he was still stuck, his father's hold over him weighing him down like an anchor. "I need to think about this. About how to move forward."

"Listen, Dad is sick and you seem tied up by him. Trust me when I tell you that will only drag you and Jack down," Mack offered. Rhett didn't disagree, but it went against years of bias he'd held against his dad. But Mack was right; since it didn't directly affect his position, he didn't see why he shouldn't accept.

"Okay. I'll take the job, but I would like to talk to you about Dad and how we can stay on the same page with him. This isn't easy for me."

"Me, neither. And, Rhett, I'm glad you and I are here. Talking about this. We should have done it years ago."

"Agreed." That much he was certain about. If only the rest was so easy.

"Anyway, congratulations on your appointment. We'll have HR do the paperwork to shift you to permanent full time if you're willing to forego the six-month original offer." Mack held out his hand for Rhett to shake, but he couldn't make the reach, not yet. Something else held him back.

"That sounds amazing. Thanks. But there's still only one position?" In all the chaos around his dad he'd neglected to ask about that. Dammit. Even when he was trying not to let his dad influence things, he was front and center.

"Yes. I have another option for Jack, if that's what you're asking."

"But HR said you took down the positions in the clinic."

"I did. Jack is perfect for the peds and OB position, so I made the decision to hire internally instead. Which means, since she's accepted, as soon as you do, you're both officially Austin Memorial employees." Mack's smile fell when Rhett didn't reply. "Aside from the hitch with Dad's involvement, I assumed you'd be happy about this, seeing as how it keeps you both here with Austin M, both doing what you're good at, and both working within two miles of one another."

Rhett was split in two. He was happy for both

of them, sure. They wouldn't be fighting over the same position, and Jack would have what she wanted—a way to take care of herself. It was perfect, really, and Mack was right. Why wasn't he celebrating?

"Can I ask what made you reconnect with Dad?" Rhett asked. It all came back to that. He had a woman pregnant with his baby and a fulfilling career in front of him and yet the anchor from his past kept him from grabbing both and running toward an amazing future.

He could see a happy life on the other end, if he could just put this behind him once and for all.

"Becoming a dad made me think about what lengths I would go to in order to make things right with my own child."

That sank in. Rhett also thought about what he needed to do to make things right with Jack. He cleared his throat.

"So you told Jack, and she accepted?" He'd know that himself if he hadn't been such a coward and had gone home.

Mack nodded. "I did. She signed the contract before she left."

She hadn't called him, hadn't texted to tell him the news. Hadn't responded to his texts to her…

What was she thinking?

It doesn't matter. You let your dad intrude, and she probably thinks you aren't going to ever be able to talk about commitment let alone actually commit to her. The curse of the Morrisons was in full swing. And you're it, buddy.

The email from his dad was small beans compared to this. God, the Morrison men really knew how to mess things up, didn't they?

"Can I take the night before I sign? I need to talk to Jack about all of this."

"Of course. And I'm glad to hear you say that. She's special, and regardless of what you decide to do with Dad or the job, I hope you two can work things out. I'm here no matter what."

"Me, too," Rhett said. Though he was happy to have his brother at his side as he walked out of Mack's office, he didn't know what "working out" would look like with her. And he'd never been more terrified.

When he finally got home, he was depleted physically and emotionally but hopeful he'd have the energy to talk to Jack and find out how she was doing. But right away, he felt…off. It only took a second to discover why.

He knew his eyes weren't failing him this time. Jack had moved out. Her books were off the one bookshelf he owned, her clothes were gone from his hangers, her floofy, smell-good bathroom products had vanished, leaving only one pathetic bar of soap by his side of the sink. The room looked bare, devoid of life.

Is this how he'd been living before she brought that light into his life? She'd added in every way to his home, his career, his heart, decorating each with color and joy.

And now everything felt beige and bland.

He sat on the bed and replayed the conversation he'd had with Mack about their father. Why was that the thought that came to him—especially because he'd tried to forget it—instead of where Jack had gotten help to move out, where she was now, and who she would live with?

Because if you think of those things, you'll go crazy, too. You made sure those aren't your problems to fix, so someone else gets to now.

He called her, but it went to voicemail.

Jack, I just heard from Mack what happened. I'm so happy you get to work at the clinic. I'm also sorry I wasn't there to talk about the job when you got the offer.

She wrote back right away.

I can't talk right now, not especially about that. I'm safe but upset and trying to figure out what comes next.

Why did you move out?

Nothing came for several minutes. "Come on," he muttered.

He voice-texted his brother that he'd like to meet with their dad and they chatted back and forth about how that could look so Mack could support the first meeting. It was time he moved on, either way. Sure, perhaps it would lead to more of the same, but maybe he'd build back some semblance of a relationship with his father and it could help him forge a stronger one with his own child.

Either way, it was worth the risk. Mack agreed and for the second time in as many days, said he was proud of Rhett. It was disorienting, but wonderful, too.

Finally, a response arrived from. It wasn't near as positive.

I didn't feel like I could come home every day and look you in the eye and not wish I was enough. That isn't fair to you; I know this wasn't your fault, that you warned me you couldn't give more when we met, but I need more from a relationship. When I'm settled, we can talk about sharing custody of the little bean. Congratulations on the job, Rhett. You deserve it.

Custody? Shit. He hadn't considered that, but it's what would happen if they didn't work out. And how could they? Yes, his feelings had wavered, but couldn't she see why? His life was a shit show right now. Why should he bring a perfect human growing his soon-to-be favorite human—or tied for first, anyway—into his life?

I'm so sorry.

There was so much more he wanted to say. He typed out something, then erased it. Before he sent off another reply, he paused. Whether he was all in or all out, it was time to make a decision.

All he could do was lay his fears at her feet and hope he was heard.

Thanks, she responded. And congratulations again on the job. You really will be wonderful.

Before he could think too much about it, he got in the car and sped off toward Jack's old apartment. He needed to talk to her face-to-face, where he couldn't hide behind a keyboard, but when he arrived, she wasn't there, either. Where else could she be?

Mack and Lainey. He dialed his brother's number and sure enough, Mack confirmed that Jack would be staying with them until she secured another place. Lainey and some nurses had helped her move in before Mack even had a chance to argue.

Sorry, Rhett. But I'll keep you posted on her health.

At least Rhett knew she was safe there. He turned around and went home, restless.

Thanks. As long as she's in good hands.

Rhett meant that, even if it killed him to not know where he and Jack were headed at the moment. He just couldn't believe they were done, but he needed to handle any obstacles that might get in his way of committing to her.

Can I get Dad's number? I think I'll see if he can meet me tomorrow and then I can sign the contract without any reservations.

You bet. Rhett got the number and sent off a request.

They agreed to meet the next day, and Rhett didn't know how he was going to wait so long. The rest of his life stood on the other end of that conversation, and it needed to go well. Leaving his pride behind was the only way he'd get what he needed and what he wanted for his growing family. He could do it. He could put aside his own resentment and show up for the family that had chosen him, even if it cost him.

He didn't even need to have the conversation for that to happen. He realized it. He had everything he needed, and there was still work to be done, but he'd do it, willingly.

Anything for Jack. He texted Lainey and Mack and drove over before he could overthink it.

Lainey answered the door when he arrived.

"She's in the back," she said, a sad smile on her face. "Good luck, and, Rhett?" He stopped and looked at her. "You'd better not break this poor girl's heart. I know where you sleep when you're on call, and I can make sure every code goes off in that room each night you're there."

He smiled wanly.

"Got it. Thanks, Lainey. And I hear congratulations are in order."

"Thanks. We went through our fair share of crap to get here, too, but I promise it's worth it on the other end."

He had to hope for the same thing, but so much depended on what the mother of his child had to say.

He found her in the back bedroom, unpacking her meager belongings into a dresser that was clearly going to be for Mack and Lainey's baby in the future. All he wanted was to give her a life where she'd never have to unpack anywhere but for vacation ever again. He wanted to be her safe haven.

That hit him with all the clarity he'd ever need.

"Jack," he whispered, going to her and putting his arms around her. "I'm so sorry I didn't come sooner. That I wasn't there to hear about the job."

She shrugged him off and his heart thumped with pain. "It's fine. That's not what I was hoping to talk to you about anyway. We always knew one of us would get the job, and I got the one I really wanted. We're where we need to be."

"I don't agree with that, Jack. Job-wise, sure. We are in good shape. But I want to be with you, not living apart."

"Being with me means more than just showing up and saying that, especially after avoiding this conversation until the jobs were distributed. You see that, right? I wanted to be chosen regardless of the jobs standing between us, and I never was."

"I did choose you. That's why I'm here—to tell you I want you to move back in. Be with me while we work this out. While I work on building a relationship with my dad."

"What will I get out of that? You thought I'd want to wait around while you decide if I'm worth making that kind of choice for? That our family is? Because I heard you loud and clear earlier, Rhett. You don't know what you want from us, but I do. And this—" she pointed back and forth between them "—isn't it. I thought you'd do anything to take this pain away," she added, her eyes misted over with hurt. "Not inflict more of it. Ignoring me wasn't fair, and I don't want to be loved like that the rest of my life. I want communication and commitment. The job fulfills me, but it doesn't matter if you couldn't see past the position to the person waiting for you on the other end."

He sighed, ran his fingers through his hair and groaned. "That's what I'm trying to say. Can't you see that? I want to be your partner, Jack. I know this is unconventional, that you and I are both coming from pasts that tried to snuff any hope of love or the future from us. But I'll work in a field picking berries if it means I get to come home to you each night."

"Will you be happy doing that, though? Resentment works both ways, Rhett, and I won't ever put myself in a position where someone else's happiness is put behind or in front of mine. That's why Orin got so horrible—he felt trapped to stay at his dead-end job so I could go to medical school and he took out his anger on my face, my body…" she sobbed. "My spirit."

"Oh, Jack. I'm so sorry. I'll never do that, though. You'll never hear me yell, never feel a hand on your body in anything other than passion or love."

"I know that, Rhett. You're a good man. But you're the same man I met, the one who, up until this morning, even, was steadfastly going after the same job I was, knowing what I have to lose. Sure I worked it out so I found something else, but if I hadn't? I think, at this point, I have to accept what you're not saying, what you are showing me, and the situation we're in as the truth. Being together is too hard, no matter how much we love each other. And I do love you, don't mistake that."

"I love you, too," he whispered. This wasn't how he saw this going. It was spiraling out of his control, and even though what she said made sense, life without her wasn't ever going to be okay. She was his person, she and the baby his people…

She turned away and he watched as all the light she'd brought to his life was removed from it and transplanted there, at Lainey and Mack's.

Being with Jack, right now anyway, was going to cause more harm than good for her, just as she'd thought. He couldn't stop the Morrison curse from claiming her, too. But he could save the woman he loved and the child from what being a Morrison meant. He just needed time to figure out how to do that, how to heal himself before he lost her for good.

It would hurt like hell to walk away from Jack and not repeat what they'd shared every night for the foreseeable future. To not wake up next to her. To not kiss her good-night and hear her laugh at one of his corny jokes. To hope for those things to happen in the near future, but trust in the uncertainty that may not work in his favor.

But it would hurt worse to have them under his own insecurities the way things were now. They would never be free to love and live the way they wanted. And Jack deserved to have that. She deserved everything.

No matter what happened with his father tomorrow, he still wanted to be a part of her life, to help raise the child they'd created together, but if she wasn't open to being his partner now that he'd let his family influence his decisions, he'd be crushed. Not that he'd blame her one bit.

"I'm sorry," he said. It wasn't an answer, but there was nothing more he could say that would make sense to her.

"Me, too," she whispered, and walked away. His heart wrenched, squeezed tight to the point he wondered if he was having another panic attack. But he breathed through it, until only a bruised, sore heart was left behind.

Hopefully some space and time to work on what he needed to fix would prove to be the best move for everyone; if not, he really didn't know what he'd do next.

God, it killed him not to be able to protect her and his child with absolute certainty. That was why he'd kept his distance from anyone in the first place—because family caused pain and their decisions couldn't be controlled.

He'd do his best to remedy this, and hope Jack would be there at the other end to see what being chosen looked like.

So, why did he feel as if he'd made the biggest mistake of his life letting her walk away?

CHAPTER TWELVE

JACK HAD SPENT the first couple weeks avoiding Rhett and now, it seemed, the roles were reversed. She'd texted him to find out how the meeting with his father had gone, and…nothing. Just a thumbs-up and smiley face emoji.

She was crushed. He hadn't said anything the other day when she'd commented that he hadn't chosen her until the jobs were distributed, and his silence had spoken volumes.

The worst part was wondering if she'd pushed him too hard, if she'd forced him to withdraw because she'd impatiently demanded they talk and define their relationship.

Ostensibly, she was aware that she was just setting boundaries about what she needed to feel loved and supported, especially coming from the tumult of the previous relationship she'd left, but he was also struggling with his own past. His dad had been manipulative, had tried to steamroll himself into Rhett's and Mack's lives. Maybe they'd get past that and find a new way forward now that things at the hospital had settled, but Jack had demanded that Rhett figure out how he felt about her instead of giving him space to process.

Yes, their conversation needed to happen, but maybe she could have given it room to breathe. What did she have to lose that she hadn't lost by shoving her emotions down his throat?

They needed to both take accountability for where they were, for what had gotten them there. And her text was an olive branch.

An olive branch he was ignoring.

What the actual hell? She was trying to be the bigger person to apologize for her role in their rift, and he'd gone radio silent for almost two straight days. Worse, he'd missed their latest OB appointment. It wasn't as if she needed him there for each one, but she did hope he'd want to be a part of their baby's life at least.

She had texted him about catching up on the appointment, namely the testing she'd do to make sure her "geriatric pregnancy" was going according to plan, but he didn't answer. When she'd asked one of the nursing staff if they'd seen him, he said, "the Morrison men were in meetings all day" and could he help her? His tone was clipped, likely a result of having to answer that same question ad nauseum. As it was, three people asked while they stood there.

"Not unless you want to know about my nuchal fold testing," she'd responded with a big smile. It wasn't her normal tack to be snarky, but she was running out of patience.

She stormed out of the ER on her way to the peds wing to check on Katie's progress and as she rounded the corner, she stopped in her tracks. Rhett was there, with Katie, both of them bent over a puzzle and engaged in clandestine-level whispering and laughter.

At Katie's door, Jack coughed to alert them to her presence. She got out her tablet and packet of boy band stickers she'd brought Katie in case Rhett got the idea she was searching him out.

"Dr. Elliot!" Katie exclaimed. "I've been waiting for you! I have so much tea for you."

"Tea? Can you have that on your diet?" Katie was on a clear liquid diet today to ensure she was ready for surgery the next morning. The surgeons were hopeful they would be able to resect all of the tumor this time based on the latest scans. It was such good news.

"It means gossip, *duh*."

Jack laughed. She'd never get a handle on the language of young people. Heck, even when she'd been a kid herself, she hadn't felt able to communicate with them in a language they understood. Her kindness and attentiveness were what made her a good peds doc if she could say such things about herself, but her attention to pop culture wasn't part of that.

The only time she'd felt seen and heard was by Rhett. Speaking of the man, she risked a glance at him, which she immediately regretted. He was sitting up straight, his lab coat and stethoscope both open across his chest, which was sheathed in a gray worsted wool sweater that hugged muscles she'd kissed and touched mere days ago.

To make matters worse, it appeared he had decided to grow a beard, which was partially filled in and trimmed to perfection. In another life, one where they'd have worked out, she'd have loved to rake her hands down his stubble and feel it for herself. Her lips, too…

"Tell me the gossip," she instructed Katie. To Rhett, she simply whispered, "What are you doing here? I've tried to text you about my testing this week."

"It's already in my schedule," he whispered back. "Sorry I missed the appointment today. It won't happen again, but it couldn't be helped."

She didn't want to know what that meant. What could be more important than his child's medical appointments? If this was any indication of how he'd be when their child was born… Especially since she'd seen the surgery board and Rhett hadn't performed any during those times.

"Shh," Katie said. "I'm talking to Dr. Elliot.

And isn't it time for that *meeting* you had?" Katie winked, and Rhett just turned bright pink and shook his head. He had *another* meeting? Sheesh. Had he become an admin since she'd left?

"I think I do. Well, thanks, Katie Rose. I liked chatting with you.

"Dr. Elliot," Rhett said, tossing one of his signature winks her way.

"Dr. Morrison," she said. God, she hoped her embarrassment at being caught ogling him didn't show as heat on her cheeks. "Good to see you. I… I hope you're okay."

"Oh, I'm better than okay." His smile said she should believe him, but what did that say about her, that he was so happy and hadn't reached out to her in days?

Ugh. Why couldn't she just accept that for whatever reason, she had a job thanks to him, and be done with the overromanticized version of loving him?

"Dr. Elliot?"

She shook her head out of the Rhett-shaped daydream she was in. "Yeah, Katie? Want to do a puzzle?"

"Maybe in a bit. I'm actually hoping you can grab that dessert," the girl said.

Jack frowned. "Katie, I'm sorry, but—"

"Dr. Elliot, it's not for me," she said, sounding

more like a teenager than the preteen she was. "Just…just get it, please."

"Okay." Jack got the box Katie pointed at and handed it to her.

"Could you open it for me? My palsy," she said, holding up her hands. They shook, but it almost looked like a manufactured effect.

"Sure." Jack opened the box and smiled. "Wow. What's this for? Did you know these are my favorite?"

"I did," Katie said, giggling and clapping her hands.

"You know how to win a girl over, don't you? What's this for, Katie?"

"Well, you told Dr. Morrison you'd name your firstborn child after him if he got you one of these, and since he thinks your baby is a girl, I asked if I could give it to you. The writing is from him, though."

"Well, that's sweet. I don't know that it's a girl, but I love the name Katie, so I'll talk to Rhett."

"He already agreed. But my name is actually Kathryn Rose, or Katie Rose."

"That's beautiful, hon."

Katie pointed to the frosting, reminding Jack to read it. "Okay, let's see what this is about." Jack looked down and tried to decipher the writing. It looked like part of the phrase was missing, but the frosting read, "Will you?"

"What—"

Katie giggled, her eyes on the door. Jack turned around and gasped. Rhett was there, on one knee, a ring box open in front of him. Instead of a ring, though, was a folded piece of paper. She opened it and read, "'Please join me in welcoming the Morrison Memorial Family Clinic to the Austin Memorial family. It will be headed by chief medical officer Rhett Morrison, and his wife, Jacqueline, will be the director of pediatrics. The twenty-bed facility won't just be staffed by Jacqueline; we'd like her to run it.'" It was signed by Rhett and Mack. And from what she saw, it wasn't the same clinic where she'd already been hired.

"It was too much to add all that on the brownie, so I put it here. The 'will you' is all-encompassing."

Was this a proposal to…to work for them? In a different job? It was a thrilling one, a dream position if she was being honest, but it wasn't what she wanted.

"Rhett, this is all well and good, but I have a job. When I wanted to talk, it was about—"

"Me not being ready to talk to you while we were still in the running for the same position. Right?" She nodded. Yeah, that summed it up. "And I am now. Hell, I was then, but just needed a moment to process how to do it right."

"I know. I'm so sorry I pushed you too quickly to make a decision—"

"No," he interrupted again. She frowned. "I don't mean to interrupt you, Jack, but I can't for a minute have you thinking you owe me any sort of apology. I could have asked for time, told you how much you meant to me, but I shrank away, afraid of my own shadow. I'm working on that but while I do, I want you to know you're all that's mattered since the day I met you. That's what you need to hear more than anything. The job is just a bonus that Mack and I think you'll be perfect for."

"Rhett," she whispered. "This clinic sounds amazing, but where is it? Don't we only have the two?"

"We did. Until I used my inheritance to purchase a third that takes peds cases in urban Austin and needs an overhaul. You can build it from the ground up, Director." She liked the sound of that, *really* liked it, but…

"What about your father?" Rhett's face didn't fall when she mentioned him, but his smile still struggled to stay bright on his face.

"We've got work to do, but we came to an understanding. He can get to know you and Kathryn Rose as long as he does so without strings attached to any of us."

"I love the name, by the way." The name sounded like spring in Austin, the best time of her life so far. "And that sounds fair as long as you're okay with that? But again, it wasn't about the job, Rhett," she admitted.

"I'm glad. And yes, I'm okay with giving the love of my life everything she's ever wanted, even if it wasn't about the job. Making sure you're happy outside our home will be necessary, too. And Mack and I agreed we could do better. You deserve this, you always have."

"I'm the—"

"Yep. The love of my life. I love you so much, Jack Elliot, that I want to be a better man for you and our daughter, or didn't you get that with the note I just gave you? I want to be a better son and brother so you have a big, happy family to come home to each night. I want to love you the rest of your life and do everything I can to give you the life you deserve, or at least get out of the way and let you help design it without my damn family getting in the way."

"Hey. That's me you're talking about."

A man walked in who looked a lot like Rhett, but shorter and stockier. He had a mischievous smile, though, which Jack had noticed was a Morrison trait.

"Jack, I'm—"

"Mr. Morrison," she said, putting down the brownie and hugging him. "Thank you for what you've done for me." The job and the clinic were almost too much. But she would appreciate both.

"My pleasure. It'll be nice having a daughter-in-law to tell me all about my son and his shenanigans."

"A daughter-in-law?" Jack asked. "Oh, Rhett and I aren't—"

"Oh yeah, that. You still haven't responded to my proposal. I guess I need to be clearer in more than one area of our romance," Rhett said, chuckling. He reached in his pocket and pulled out a gold and diamond-encrusted ring that shone in the mediocre hospital lighting. "Will you marry me? Be my partner in every sense of the word? This isn't at all related to the job, though I do hope you'll be willing to coordinate our schedules so we can spend every available moment outside of work together."

Jack hadn't realized she'd begun crying until the vision of the ring blurred. She was nodding and wiping away tears while Katie whooped in the background.

Thankfully, her vision cleared enough to see him slip the ring on her finger where it sparkled and made all the sense in the world.

"Yes," Jack whispered. "I'd love to marry you, Rhett. I love you so much." She glanced down at the ring and the arrow tattoo that now pointed at her future, her love, her Rhett.

"I love you, too, Jack. More than yesterday and less than tomorrow."

They kissed and Jack knew with absolute certainty that yes, indeed, everything would be okay. In fact, it would be better than anything she could have ever imagined.

EPILOGUE

RHETT TURNED AND pressed a kiss to the shoulder of the woman standing next to him. Her skin was warm from the sun pouring over them during their kid-free kayak excursion. He loved the insider knowledge that she was more than a little sun-kissed in places no one could see at that moment, but that he'd been lucky enough to enjoy earlier. They'd pulled over in the mangroves and found a small stretch of beach where he'd made love to his wife. God, he loved Jack.

Everything about her made him better—from her gentle guidance through his reconciliation with his father, never pushing but always curious to her mothering of their almost-toddler. Jack was the best mother to Kathryn Rose, and he hoped they'd be lucky enough on this family vacation to add to that joy by giving their daughter a sibling.

"She's so cute when she does that," Jack said, nuzzling into the nook of Rhett's shoulder.

Their daughter, Kathryn Rose, splashed in the

shallow end of the resort pool, laughing each time she sprayed herself with the warm water.

"I love that giggle. I hope she never outgrows it," he added. She was named after Katie who'd been instrumental in getting his wife not only the double-thick frosted brownie she'd joked about when they first met, but her agreeing to marry him.

Speaking of the original Katie, she had also walked as the flower girl in his and Jack's wedding last year, pushing Kathryn Rose in her stroller. Katie's tumor was no longer growing, and though she would need to keep an eye on it the rest of her life, she was back to living the childhood she'd always dreamed about. But not before she got to see her favorite British boy band in concert as a gift from Rhett and Jack for being in the wedding.

"What do you want to do for dinner, Dr. Morrison?" Jack asked. He not-so-secretly loved when she called him that. Especially when they got to work the same shift at the clinic.

"Up to you, Dr. Morrison," he teased, kissing her forehead. As much as he loved hearing her call him Dr. Morrison, he especially loved saying it back to her for all it implied—mostly that she was leaving her awful past behind her and starting a future with him. "I think we should get a sitter and enjoy this last evening together."

"Oh, yeah? What do you have in mind, husband?"

She reached up on her toes and kissed him. One of his favorite things about loving this woman was watching how alive she'd become with the love they shared. She flirted, had started letting loose with singing and dancing at home both with and without Kathryn Rose, and she'd ventured out to find a group of friends who had a book club together. It had been a rocky start for him and Jack, but she'd been patient as he worked through his challenges, and now they were as strong and formidable a couple as ever.

"I think a good bottle of wine is in order," he said, kissing her softly on the lips. "And then a lobster dinner by the waterfront." She moaned as he kissed beneath her ear. He didn't care who saw.

"Then what?"

"Oh, I have plans for you that involve coconut oil, a bed and you, naked. Let's just leave it at that." He pulled her into him and kissed her deeply. "I love you, Jack Morrison," he whispered.

"I love you, too, Rhett. More than yesterday and not as much as tomorrow."

They kissed as their daughter giggled, cheering them on in her own playful way. Life may have been an adventure leading up to Rhett and Jack's auspicious start, but it was nothing compared to the one ahead of them. It wasn't a racetrack, or a rodeo arena, but something even better. It was the adventure of loving and being loved in return and that was all Rhett would ever need.

* * * * *

If you missed the previous story in the Paging Dr. Morrison duet, then check out Expecting in ER *by Tina Beckett*

And if you enjoyed this story, check out these other great reads from Kristine Lynn

Wedding Date with Dr. Petrides
How to Resist Your Enemy
Nine Months to Marry the Princess

All available now!